Promoting Child AND Parent Wellbeing

How to Use Evidence- and Strengths-Based Strategies in Practice

Carole Sutton

Jessica Kingsley *Publishers*
London and Philadelphia

First published in 2016
by Jessica Kingsley Publishers
73 Collier Street
London N1 9BE, UK
and
400 Market Street, Suite 400
Philadelphia, PA 19106, USA

www.jkp.com

Library of Congress Cataloging in Publication Data

Sutton, Carole, author.
  Promoting child and parent wellbeing : how to use evidence- and strengths-based strategies in practice
/ Carole Sutton.
     pages cm
  Includes bibliographical references.
  ISBN 978-1-84905-572-7 (alk. paper)
  1. Family social work--Great Britain. 2. Social work with children--Great Britain. 3. Child welfare--Great
Britain. 4. Child development--Great Britain. 5. Parents--Services for--Great Britain. 6. Children--
Services for--Great Britain. I. Title.
  HV700.G7S87 2016
  362.71'6--dc23
                                        2015031253

British Library Cataloguing in Publication Data
A CIP catalogue record for this book is available from the British Library

ISBN 978 1 84905 572 7
eISBN 978 1 78450 015 3

Printed and bound in Great Britain

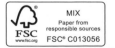

To all volunteers who give so generously of their time and energies to helping so many people in our communities, but whose contributions often go unnoticed. In warm appreciation...

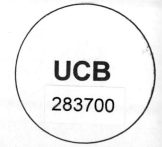

Acknowledgements

I should like to thank several people who have helped me with the preparation of this book: Hellmuth Weich and Elis King both read early drafts and made extremely useful suggestions; Jane Petrie brought very relevant research studies to my attention and Rohit Taylor and Aatif Patel at De Montfort University were both very helpful in tracing references and procedures for me. I am very grateful to them all.

Contents

Facilitating close relationships with nurseries, playgroups
and schools

The helping person as positive model, coach and architect
of success

Introduction

OVERVIEW

- So what do we mean by children's wellbeing?
- Early intervention to support families is essential
- Some policy initiatives by central government
- A matrix of cumulative risk and protective factors
- Values, knowledge and skills for practice
- A chronological focus and the evidence selected
- A process for practice: ASPIRE
- The Common Assessment Framework (CAF)

I find it deeply satisfying to be writing this book at a time when the focus on risks and difficulties encountered by children and young people is gradually being be replaced by a focus on their strengths and resilience and on factors which offer them protection. It is high time!

SO WHAT DO WE MEAN BY CHILDREN'S WELLBEING?

In September 2013, the National Institute for Health and Care Excellence (NICE) issued a Local Government Briefing on Social and Emotional Wellbeing for Children and Young People, stating that it 'laid the foundations for healthy behaviours and educational attainment. It also helps prevent behavioural problems (including substance misuse) and mental health problems.' Definitions are shown in Box I.1.

> **Box I.1 Definitions of emotional, psychological and social wellbeing (NICE 2013)**
>
> - *Emotional wellbeing:* This includes being happy and self-confident and not anxious or depressed.
>
> - *Psychological wellbeing:* This includes the ability to be autonomous, problem-solve, manage emotions, experience empathy, and be resilient and attentive.
>
> - *Social wellbeing:* Has good relationships with others, and does not have behavioural problems; that is, not disruptive, violent or bullying.

Children's and young people's mental health

Although the main focus of this book will be on positive features of children's and young people's development, we must acknowledge such data as are available concerning their mental health at the present time. The recent NHS England Review (NHS England 2014, p.15) is still based on out-of-date information:

> The best available estimates of the prevalence of mental disorders among children and young people are those from the Office for National Statistics surveys in 1999 and 2004. These found that one in ten children aged between five and sixteen years has a mental disorder. About half of these (5.8%) have a conduct disorder, 3.7% an emotional disorder (anxiety, depression), 1–2% have severe Attention Deficit Hyperactivity Disorder (ADHD) and 1% have neurodevelopmental disorders. The rates of disorder rise steeply in middle to late adolescence...

Further, in 2011 the Department for Education had reported that over 50 per cent of UK children starting formal education (typically at five years of age) were considered not to be 'school ready'. That is, they lacked sufficient physical, social, emotional, cognitive or language skills to access the learning set out in the Key Stage 1 curriculum. Moreover, the important Allen Report, entitled *Early Intervention: The Next Steps*, published in the same year as an independent report to government, reiterated the case for early intervention to support young children and their parents, with several startling illustrations from the research literature (Box I.2).

Box I.2 Examples of links between early experience and later outcomes (Allen Report 2011, p.xiii)

- A child's development score at just 22 months can serve as an accurate predictor of educational outcomes at 26 years.

- Some 54 per cent of the incidents of depression in women and 58 per cent of suicide attempts by women have been attributed to adverse childhood experiences, according to a study in the USA.

- An authoritative study of boys assessed by nurses at age three as being 'at risk' found that they had two-and-a-half times as many criminal convictions as the group deemed not to be at risk at age 21. Moreover, in the at-risk group, 55 per cent of the convictions were for violent offences, compared with 1 per cent for those who were deemed not to be at risk.

The report continues, using evidence in the public domain, to insist upon the case for early intervention to support families. So in these depressing circumstances what use can we make of relevant research evidence in order to respond constructively?

EARLY INTERVENTION TO SUPPORT FAMILIES IS ESSENTIAL

While it was essential and appropriate that researchers in psychology and other social sciences should initially examine risks and hazards for children's difficulties in great depth, both to identify them and to pinpoint the links between these risks and mental ill health, school failure and offending, much of this work has now been done – by, for example, Robins (1966), Patterson (1976) and Moffitt (1993).

So now, with much of this knowledge extant, researchers are beginning to focus on *the positive factors and practices* which protect children and young people from encountering and succumbing to the risks posed by disadvantage and a range of threats and hazards. Within the social sciences, for example, we have Carr's *Positive Psychology:*

The Science of Happiness and Human Strengths (2004) while within social work we have Saleebey's *The Strengths Perspective in Social Work Practice* (2005).

A most important publication is *The Signs of Safety: Child Protection Practice Framework* (Government of Western Australia 2011). Within this, practitioners have first to document what they are worried about in a family situation where a child's safety is at issue, but are then required specifically to identify '*What's working well?*' They then have to go on to make absolutely clear what needs to happen to keep the child safe. These and similar publications with their emphasis on strengths rather than problems guide us to look at mental *health*, not *ill health*, at a family's achievements rather than its shortcomings, and at discipline and prosocial behaviour in young people rather than at patterns of delinquency and offending.

I repeat my gladness that I am alive at such a time, when after centuries of blame and condemnation of difficult children and young people it is becoming evident that a focus on their strengths and their positive features can often completely turn round situations which seemed to promise nothing but failure, distress and misery. And that is true for their parents and other adults too!

But the work has to begin early. While such aphorisms as 'The child is father of the man' and 'Give me a child until he is seven and I will give you the man' have alerted us through the ages to the existence of a link between childhood and adult experience, it is only within the last few decades that there have been the beginnings of a rigorous evidence base in this field.

There has been much research attention devoted to the phenomenon of *attachment*, the intimate emotional relationship which normally develops between an infant and his or her main carer, usually the mother but whoever gives the baby the most sustained and regular care and attention. The term 'attachment' is usually used to describe the link between infant and caregiver; the link between caregiver and infant is usually called 'bonding'. These relationships seem to underpin the wellbeing, not only of the developing infant but also of the mother, father and all those who care for the child.

As we shall see, it was the work of, among others, John Bowlby and his team, of which a notable member was Mary Ainsworth (see

Ainsworth *et al.* 1978), that drew attention to the impact of early experience upon subsequent adult lives. We shall explore this work in some detail. Since then, literally hundreds of studies, reports and publications have focused on the vulnerability of troubled children and their families. Follow-up studies, for example by Lyons-Ruth (1996), have shown that children deprived of a reliable, warm and loving relationship with one or more adults committed to their welfare are far more likely to become unhappy and troubled children. Many studies have documented the evidence that serious misbehaviour, tantrums, defiance, persistent verbal or physical aggression by children in the early years of their lives presages convictions for offending in adulthood (for example, Fergusson, Horwood and Ridder 2005).

I remember my own startled reaction when, embarking on the literature search for my PhD research, I encountered the paper by Stevenson and Goodman (2001) entitled 'Association between behaviour at age 3 years and adult criminality'. Before that time, such a link had never crossed my mind. Now at last, however, we can begin to offer effective interventions at these early stages which may strengthen positive behaviours and provide a trajectory away from, rather than towards, adult criminality.

SOME POLICY INITIATIVES BY CENTRAL GOVERNMENT

As the evidence of the early origins of many children's difficulties filtered through to central government and to the policy-making bodies, major initiatives have been taken. For example, in 1995 Child and Adolescent Mental Health (CAMHS) teams were established throughout the country to provide urgently needed services for supporting children and their families, while in 1997 a major review of services for young children and their families, which cut across government departments, was undertaken. This led to the opening of the first Sure Start centres in a number of disadvantaged localities in Britain. The centres were to provide early education for preschool children, integrated with health and family-support services and extended childcare services. Control of the centres was to be exercised through local partnerships among professionals, voluntary organisations, health visitors and a wide forum of other practitioners. Latterly, there is a requirement that a qualified teacher shall be involved in developing the curriculum and the day-to-day programme for the children. Practice must be evidence based and support for parents must be readily available.

Sure Start centres were eventually built or developed throughout England. There were subsequently slightly different versions in Scotland, Wales and Northern Ireland.

They are now typically called Sure Start Children's Centres, or in some localities Children, Young People and Families Centres. Their work contributed to the strategic objectives of *Every Child Matters*, the major central government policy document published in 2003 by the Department for Education. This concerns all children from birth to age 19 and aims to improve educational achievement and reduce the levels of ill health, teenage pregnancy, child abuse and neglect as well as crime and antisocial behaviour. The main aims of this initiative, details of which are now enshrined in the Children Act 2004, are for all children to have the support they need to achieve the outcomes set out in *Every Child Matters* and listed in Box I.3.

Box I.3 The five outcomes set out in
Every Child Matters **(2003)**

- Stay safe
- Be healthy
- Enjoy and achieve
- Make a positive contribution
- Achieve economic wellbeing.

Each of the themes is embedded in a detailed framework of practice to be observed by multi-agency partnerships in collaboration (see Cheminais 2009).

The impact of such investment has been evaluated on several occasions, and in 2008 an inquiry into the Sure Start Local Programme (SSLP) found that children living in several SSLP areas, by comparison with those living in similar areas but without SSLP provision, demonstrated the following (National Evaluation of Sure Start Research Team 2008):

- Parents of three-year-old children showed less negative parenting while providing their children with a better home learning environment.

- Three-year-old children in SSLP areas had higher levels of positive social behaviour and independence/self-regulation than children in similar areas not having an SSLP.

- The SSLP effects for positive social behaviour appeared to be a consequence of the SSLP positive benefits upon parenting.

While ongoing funding for such Children's Centres is far from certain, the government has placed emphasis on the crucial role played by parents in protecting their young children from difficulties and enhancing their development, and has made funds available for the establishing of parenting programmes – packages of knowledge and skills which can be taught to parents by carefully trained practitioners.

Additionally, programmes such as The Incredible Years (Webster-Stratton 1992), Triple P (Sanders 1999) and Strengthening Families, Strengthening Communities (Steele *et al.* 1999) have all been rigorously evaluated and have for the most part shown many benefits in helping parents to manage their children's difficulties and enrich their development. However, people who wish to use these resources are required to attend extensive courses of training and to keep demonstrating their commitment to 'treatment fidelity' – in other words, that they are faithfully following the detailed steps in which they were trained and are not introducing sequences from other trainings to which they themselves are particularly attached.

Although these programmes, employing highly experienced trainers, have repeatedly demonstrated excellent outcomes, they are very costly indeed and are often beyond the resources of health authorities and departments of social service. In these circumstances practitioners are thrown back on parenting training and resources which have worked well for them in the past – even though they may not have demonstrated outcomes at the most rigorous statistical level. Experienced practitioners using these alternative ways of working with parents have been able to demonstrate outcomes which satisfy parents' immediate needs: children sleep, they comply with requests, they cease to be aggressive and hard to manage and often become settled and pleasant to be with; parents commend and praise their children, they spend more time with them, ignore mild misbehaviour and are consistent in penalising more serious misbehaviour; younger children even begin to demonstrate levels of attachment to their parents which delight all who know them (Sutton 2006).

So in times of austerity, what can hard-pressed practitioners do? We suggest they can learn from all that research has revealed about protective factors for children, and at whatever stage in the life cycle that they encounter a child and his or her family they can draw on those research findings for practice. We shall consider many of these findings below.

It is important to make clear that this book is not primarily concerned with child protection: rather it is hoped that it will make a contribution towards safeguarding children. Brayne and Carr (2008) explain: 'Safeguarding and promoting the welfare of children is not statutorily defined. However, it is a crucial term within the Children Act 2004 which is intended to have wide application. It is distinct from the notion of child protection which is key to the Children Act 1989… Child protection is linked to legally based state intervention; safeguarding is a means of ensuring that children receive the support they need for their well-being.' A closely associated publication is *Working Together to Safeguard Children. A Guide to Inter-Agency Working to Safeguard and Promote the Welfare of Children* (Department for Education 2015) which recently updated the report of the same name published two years earlier. A further very important relevant publication is *The Healthy Child Programme*, which, first published in 2009, is regularly updated. The current version is entitled *Rapid Review to Update Evidence for the Healthy Child Programme 0–5* (Public Health England 2015).

A MATRIX OF CUMULATIVE RISK AND PROTECTIVE FACTORS

In order to accommodate the array of interacting variables which impinge on children and their parents, two colleagues and I prepared a matrix of factors displaying these – according to the age of the child. This matrix is shown in Figure I.1 (Sutton, Utting and Farrington 2004).

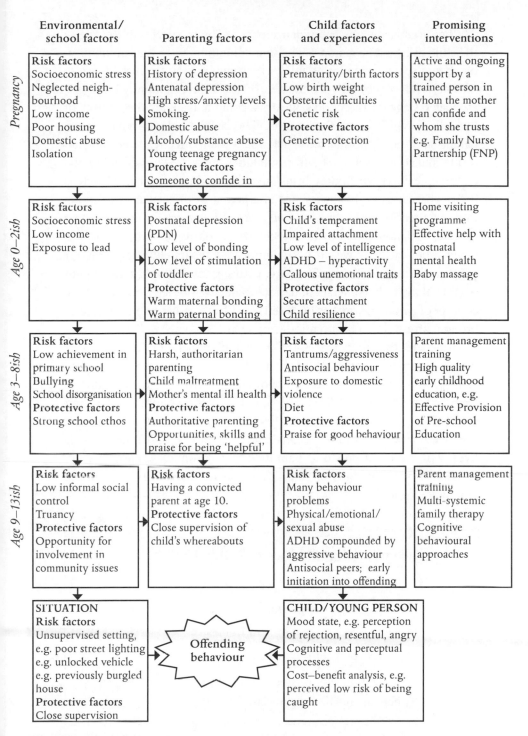

Environmental/ school factors	Parenting factors	Child factors and experiences	Promising interventions
Pregnancy **Risk factors** Socioeconomic stress Neglected neigh- bourhood Low income Poor housing Domestic abuse Isolation	**Risk factors** History of depression Antenatal depression High stress/anxiety levels Smoking. Domestic abuse Alcohol/substance abuse Young teenage pregnancy **Protective factors** Someone to confide in	**Risk factors** Prematurity/birth factors Low birth weight Obstetric difficulties Genetic risk **Protective factors** Genetic protection	Active and ongoing support by a trained person in whom the mother can confide and whom she trusts e.g. Family Nurse Partnership (FNP)
Age 0–2ish **Risk factors** Socioeconomic stress Low income Exposure to lead	**Risk factors** Postnatal depression (PDN) Low level of bonding Low level of stimulation of toddler **Protective factors** Warm maternal bonding Warm paternal bonding	**Risk factors** Child's temperament Impaired attachment Low level of intelligence ADHD – hyperactivity Callous unemotional traits **Protective factors** Secure attachment Child resilience	Home visiting programme Effective help with postnatal mental health Baby massage
Age 3–8ish **Risk factors** Low achievement in primary school Bullying School disorganisation **Protective factors** Strong school ethos	**Risk factors** Harsh, authoritarian parenting Child maltreatment Mother's mental ill health **Protective factors** Authoritative parenting Opportunities, skills and praise for being 'helpful'	**Risk factors** Tantrums/aggressiveness Antisocial behaviour Exposure to domestic violence Diet **Protective factors** Praise for good behaviour	Parent management training High quality early childhood education, e.g. Effective Provision of Pre-school Education
Age 9–13ish **Risk factors** Low informal social control Truancy **Protective factors** Opportunity for involvement in community issues	**Risk factors** Having a convicted parent at age 10. **Protective factors** Close supervision of child's whereabouts	**Risk factors** Many behaviour problems Physical/emotional/ sexual abuse ADHD compounded by aggressive behaviour Antisocial peers; early initiation into offending	Parent management training Multi-systemic family therapy Cognitive behavioural approaches
SITUATION **Risk factors** Unsupervised setting, e.g. poor street lighting e.g. unlocked vehicle e.g. previously burgled house **Protective factors** Close supervision	**Offending behaviour**	**CHILD/YOUNG PERSON** Mood state, e.g. perception of rejection, resentful, angry Cognitive and perceptual processes Cost–benefit analysis, e.g. perceived low risk of being caught	

Figure I.1 Risk, protection and prevention
Reproduced, with updates, from Sutton et al. (2004). Reproduced under the terms of the Open Government Licence v2.0.

All the variables shown are evidence based. The rows refer to the age of the child as he or she matures. The first column refers to the community-based and socioeconomic variables which impinge on families: housing, income, levels of supportive contact with others and community resources; at a later stage in the child's life this column includes the impact of the school which he or she attends. The second column refers to the parents and the circumstances which affect them directly: health, mental health and relationships. The third includes characteristics of individual children, features which they bring into the world with them, as well as their experiences as they grow up. The layout of the matrix is intended to draw attention to the *ways in which variables interact*; for example, low income, isolation, poor maternal health, smoking in pregnancy and many other factors have all been implicated separately as hazards for subsequent child wellbeing in different studies, but these hazards do not operate alone – they interact and 'potentiate' each other. So recently the concept of *cumulative risk* has been retrieved from earlier publications and brought afresh to public attention (Appleyard *et al.* 2005).

One of the first pieces of research which highlighted this phenomenon of cumulative risk was the now classic Isle of Wight/ Central London borough study conducted by Michael Rutter and his team and published in 1978. This compared the children and young people living in these two very different communities and identified a number of risk factors for emotional and behavioural difficulties in their lives. The team developed a 'Family Adversity Index' comprising six stressors which impinged on families: these are listed in Box I.4 in the language of the day.

Box I.4 Family Adversity Index (Rutter 1978)

1. Father: unskilled/semiskilled job

2. Overcrowding or large family size ['large' was not defined]

3. Marital discord and/or broken home

4. Mother: depression/neurosis

5. Child ever 'in care'

6. Father: any offence against law.

The team found that children living in London with only one family stressor did not pose any particular risk for subsequent difficulties, poor mental health, poor experience at school or becoming an offender, but if a child experienced two stressors the risk increased fourfold, while if there were four stressors the risk rose tenfold. Comparison children living in the Isle of Wight experienced much lower levels of risk. Other researchers have used somewhat different risk factors from those identified by Rutter, but have found the same process of increasing risk as the number of stressors accumulated: children with accumulating high risks had dramatically poorer outcomes than those with few risks. As Appleyard *et al.* (2005) summarise this concept: 'The findings support the cumulative risk hypothesis that the number of risks in early childhood predicts behaviour problems in adolescence...' but, they continue: 'The results support the need for comprehensive prevention and early intervention efforts with high-risk children, such as there does not appear to be a point beyond which services for children are hopeless.' The authors go on to say that reducing any risk factor makes a difference. This principle is the central underpinning theme for this book: moreover, it focuses not primarily on reducing risk factors but on strengthening protective factors affecting children.

I would encourage you to reflect on this matrix at the end of each chapter as you read through the book.

VALUES, KNOWLEDGE AND SKILLS FOR PRACTICE

Values which underpin ethical and professional practice

Whether it is delivered by psychologists, social workers, health visitors, probation officers, members of the medical professions or volunteers, help is offered within a framework of values and ethics. I give in Box I.5 the value base of helping families with troubled children published in an earlier book (Sutton 2006).

Box 1.5 The value base of helping families with troubled children

1. All children and young people are intrinsically valuable. They are to be cared for and respected.

2. The overall aim of the work is to enable parents to continue to care for their children.

3. Diverse family patterns are to be acknowledged and respected.

4. Cultural diversity is to be acknowledged and respected.

5. Each child is unique, with a unique history and background.

6. Families benefit from being respected and empowered.

7. Parents' existing strengths, knowledge and experience should be built upon.

8. Practice must be actively anti-discriminatory.

9. The involvement of fathers and grandparents as well as mothers in promoting their children's welfare is invaluable.

10. Children are the responsibility of the wider society as well as of their families.

In particular, practitioners, whatever their background, must practise in an anti-discriminatory way, offering all those with whom they come into contact knowledge and skills according to their needs. Thompson (2006) has made an analysis of the circumstances of many of those with whom social practitioners work by highlighting how 'inequalities and discrimination feature in the social circumstances of clients, and in the interactions between clients and the welfare state, it is helpful to analyse the situation in terms of three levels'; these three levels are known as the PCS analysis (Box I.6).

> **Box 1.6 The PCS analysis of discrimination (Thompson 2006)**
>
> - P refers to the *personal* or *psychological* – the individual level of thoughts, feelings, attitudes and actions. It also refers to *practice*, individual workers interacting with individual clients, and *prejudice*, the inflexibility of mind which stands in the way of fair and non-judgemental practice ...
> - C refers to the *cultural* levels of shared ways of seeing, thinking and doing. It relates to the *commonalities* – values and patterns of thought and behaviour, an assumed *consensus* about what is right and what is normal; it produces *conformity* to social norms ...
> - S refers to the *structural* level, the network of *social divisions* and the power relations that are so closely associated with them; it also refers to the ways in which oppression and discrimination are institutionalised and thus *'sewn in'* to the fabric of society ...

Thompson quotes Berger (1966, p.140) on how we internalise, take into ourselves, the social values and cultural norms of the societies in which we live:

> Society not only controls our movements, but shapes our identity, our thoughts and our emotions. The structures of society become the structure of our own consciousness. Society does not stop at the surface of our skins. Society penetrates us as much as it envelops us.

Thompson goes on to urge that we as practitioners, whose activities may profoundly affect the lives of others, should become aware of our own enculturation, and should through self-reflection and in the course of supervision become alert to how our own personal beliefs, acquired from our cultures and norms, may be negatively impacting on those whom we claim to be helping. Such reflective practice can both raise our own awareness and identify ways of building the confidence and self-esteem of people who have been battered by life but who with our support and encouragement can renew their efforts to tackle the challenges and difficulties which they encounter.

Knowledge from research which can inform practice

I am writing this book because of the amount and importance of the research directly affecting practice which is continuing to pour out from universities, colleges, hospitals and schools. When I trained as a medical social worker many years ago on a one-year course at the London School of Economics I was given a brief course of lectures on psychoanalytic and psychodynamic theory, and another on social administration, and then, armed with these ideas and a certain amount of common sense, I was let loose on the public. I am not at all sure that I did no harm, but I was fortunate to have some excellent practice tutors and other colleagues along the way through whom I learned about empirical research and what could be learned through applying these principles.

Since then, many, many bodies of theory have been formalised, and this book will draw to readers' attention some of the central ones, now established by large bodies of evidence, which must inform practice: attachment theory, the concepts of client-centred practice, social learning theory, cognitive behavioural theory and motivational interviewing (MI). Inevitably, in a short book such as this, the concepts cannot be explored in depth, but the key principles will be set out for readers to take further. Now, some years later, and with several years of research and teaching within psychology behind me, I am still learning from almost every research paper I read. As the demands on practitioners become ever greater, so the standards and amount of research are increasing. What we really need are the resources to disseminate and make use of the research evidence.

Skills to inform practice

We know a good deal about key skills of working with people – for example, that of forming positive relationships – and we have done so since at least the middle years of the last century. In 1951 Carl Rogers published his seminal text, *Client-Centred Therapy*, and while we are here concerned with helping and supporting people, not with therapy, it is clear that one of the key principles identified by Rogers, namely demonstrating 'unconditional positive regard' for all whom we encounter, is fundamental to all helping relationships. A few years later, in 1967, Truax and Carkfuff published another seminal text of direct relevance to the skills of building positive relationships, *Towards Effective Counselling and Psychotherapy*. This huge study, underpinned by rigorous research, showed that it was not so much the theoretical position of the counsellor that brought about greater wellbeing and 'improvement' on the part of clients. Rather it was whether the counsellor or therapist brought to bear three specific ways of interacting with clients: *empathy* for the person concerned in his or her circumstances, *respectful warmth* and *genuineness* – an authentic as distinct from a feigned manner of interaction.

While, as we shall see, other researchers have brought further bodies of ideas to inform theories of working with those in distress or in need of help, no constellation of ideas has, to the best of my knowledge, supplanted the principles of unconditional positive regard, conveyed by empathy, warmth and genuineness. We shall explore these further in Chapter 1, on pregnancy.

A CHRONOLOGICAL FOCUS AND THE EVIDENCE SELECTED

The book follows a chronological sequence, considering the risks and protective factors which affect a child as he or she, surrounded by family, friends and community, matures and develops. We shall begin in pregnancy where already certain genetically endowed features and environmental influences are exerting their influence and which both directly and indirectly affect the child's life chances and potentials for good or ill. We shall consider how it is essential for the helping person to establish warm and empathic relationships with those whom they are trying to support and how those relationships carry huge influence for good. We shall explore principles of 'motivational interviewing' and see how we may draw on them to help pregnant mothers and their partners to consider their ongoing patterns of smoking or alcohol or substance use. We shall see how processes of bonding between mother and baby can begin during this amazing period.

In Chapter 2, on birth and the first year of life, we shall see how helpers can assist families who have just come through the extraordinary experience of childbirth, and help a new baby to get off to a good start. So we shall consider the evidence concerning key features of the parent–child relationship, breastfeeding, helping establish routines of sleeping and feeding and father involvement. We shall consider the work of Brazelton and Nugent (1995) and see how sensitive carers can help parents to discern their baby's preferences for light or dark at different times of day, for activity or calm, and for times for sleeping or times of interaction with them. Later, we shall explore how it is possible to support mothers and fathers in bonding with their new baby and then, later in that first year, how the natural processes of attachment by the baby to key people in his world can be recognised and facilitated. We shall also consider postnatal depression (PND) and the evidence for several means of assisting mothers and fathers to deal with this, including active listening, medication and cognitive behavioural therapy (CBT). Some key concepts from CBT will be briefly introduced.

In Chapter 3, concerning the child aged one to two years, we shall focus on the need to encourage the development of bonding and attachment, while helping all those who care for the child to establish sensitive yet confident and authoritative parenting. We shall explore the characteristics of such parenting and show that while any word which includes the stem 'authority' may offend families who believe that all that is needed to bring up a child is love, a healthy attention to setting boundaries for a child and perhaps, surprisingly, to help them to begin to develop self-control, even at this young age, are valuable foundations for later life.

In Chapter 4, concerning the ages three to eight, we shall follow the child into the world of school and explore how families can prepare him or her for that. We shall examine the particular experiences which help to equip the child for the hurly-burly of the school playground and how authoritative parenting continues to offer support and protection throughout this period. We shall explore play and language in some detail, showing that good preschool education can compensate for a wide range of limited experiences or total omissions in a child's early life and how stories and an array of play activities are invaluable in helping a child reach his or her cognitive potential.

In Chapter 5, concerning the years nine to thirteen, as the child matures and comes increasingly under the influence of groups of other children, we shall explore the necessity of close supervision of his or her activities. We shall show how it is invaluable for the child and parent(s) to share interests and enthusiasms, for him or her to be able to accompany members of the family to their interests and activities, so that there is a strong foundation of family cohesion and shared experience contributing to the child's development. We shall reiterate the usefulness of parenting management skills training, so that families can learn from the array of research which has been carried out how they can appreciate their child, encourage the child and guide him or her with an authoritative, but not authoritarian, style. We shall look too at the major contribution which many schools make towards building supportive home/school relationships, where parents see the school as engaged in a joint initiative to enable each child to develop and flourish.

Chapter 6 comprises a brief summary and recapitulation of key ideas and principles for encouraging parents and their young children.

Wherever possible, I have referred to rigorously designed studies – in most cases randomised controlled trials (RCTs) and well-established bodies of evidence. For example, the studies which were examined by Truax and Carkhuff (1967), already mentioned, when exploring the impact of a range of approaches found helpful and effective to those receiving counselling, were exhaustively statistically analysed before conclusions were drawn. The evidence of the quality of this research is that it has never been convincingly challenged and to the best of my knowledge it underpins all approaches to helping people in distress which have been developed since. Similarly, the important work of the team supporting The Incredible Years parenting package used and uses RCTs routinely. For it is only by researchers repeatedly employing the highest standards of experimental design and comparing their findings with those of others who use similar high standards that it is possible to state that the evidence supports or does not support a claim. For example, we can now claim with considerable confidence that harsh parenting is one of the variables which contributes to major difficulties in the lives of children born to those parents. We shall explore this evidence as we proceed.

A PROCESS FOR PRACTICE: ASPIRE

In an earlier book, *Helping Families with Troubled Children* (Sutton 2006), I introduced the mnemonic ASPIRE, which seems to have been found useful as a means of conceptualising the processes of practice by a number of professional groups. For example, I understand that probation officers are trained to use this sequence as a framework for thinking about the process of their practice. The letters of the mnemonic stand for stages of the process as listed in Box I.7 and illustrated in Figure I.2.

**Box I.7 The ASPIRE process
(after Sutton and Herbert 1992)**

AS   Assessment

P   Planning

I   Implementation of the plan

R   Review

E   Evaluation

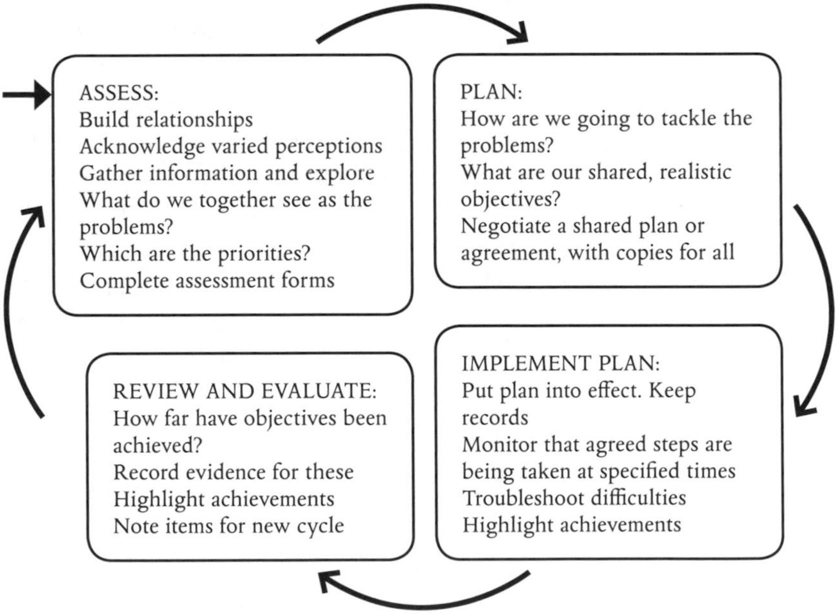

ASSESS:
Build relationships
Acknowledge varied perceptions
Gather information and explore
What do we together see as the problems?
Which are the priorities?
Complete assessment forms

PLAN:
How are we going to tackle the problems?
What are our shared, realistic objectives?
Negotiate a shared plan or agreement, with copies for all

REVIEW AND EVALUATE:
How far have objectives been achieved?
Record evidence for these
Highlight achievements
Note items for new cycle

IMPLEMENT PLAN:
Put plan into effect. Keep records
Monitor that agreed steps are being taken at specified times
Troubleshoot difficulties
Highlight achievements

Figure I.2 *The ASPIRE process as a cycle*

THE COMMON ASSESSMENT FRAMEWORK (CAF)

The ASPIRE process is used of course in association with the CAF, which is used by practitioners across Britain. Although there have been variants developed in different localities, the CAF remains the underpinning framework for all assessments of children in need of help (Figure I.3) and investigates the following three fields:

- The child's developmental needs, including whether they are suffering or likely to suffer significant harm

- Parents' or carers' capacity to respond to those needs

- The impact and influence of wider family, community and environmental circumstances.

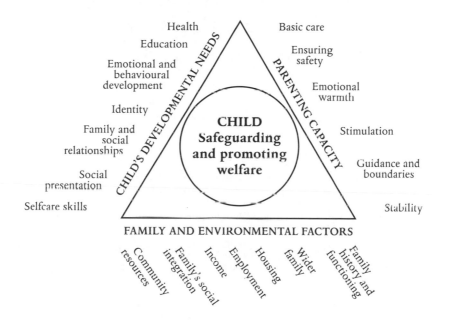

Figure I.3 *The Common Assessment Framework (Department of Health 2000)*

While practitioners focusing on children's wellbeing are not likely to be called upon to make assessments as full as those indicated by the CAF, they should nevertheless be aware that these are the variables and factors which contribute to the family's, and thus the child's, wellbeing. They may well have their own observations to add to those of other practitioners.

There have inevitably been developments concerning the completion of so lengthy an assessment tool as the CAF, and in some parts of the country, for example Bristol, a Single Assessment Framework (SAF) (Box I.8) is emerging, which merits attention as it may be of use to a range of practitioners. The authorities write: 'This multi-agency assessment allows professionals working with a family to have a shared understanding of the families' strengths and what support they need to thrive. It will mean that families don't have to experience multiple assessments undertaken by a wide variety of professionals... We have replaced the Common Assessment Framework (CAF) in Bristol as the early help assessment, with the SAF.'

Box I.8 Levels of assessment offered in the Single Assessment Framework (Bristol)

- *Initial contact.* A Request for Help form is used when a child and/or a family are first identified as requiring additional support.
- *SAF assessment.* The holistic assessment that provides a clear record of the different needs for a child and family ... and whether a specialist assessment is necessary.
- *Additional assessment.* Specific specialist assessments of a child where more detail is required in specific areas for more complex needs: for example speech and language, occupational therapy or psychological assessment. This includes an Education, Health and Care Plan.

It is reported that each of the three Bristol teams has an Early Help Team with specific practitioners to coordinate requests for help to support vulnerable children, young people and their families. Information gathered via the SAF is, in due course, entered onto a computer program called the Coordinating Children's System, so that appropriate practitioners can both enter and inform themselves of changes in the circumstances of children and families for and to whom they are accountable. It seems likely that similar models of coordinated information gathering and recording will lead to more effective help being made available to families in need.

This book is written for anyone who may wonder what rigorous research suggests about ways of helping families with young children – with an emphasis on building on their strengths, rather than focusing on their deficiencies. I hope it will appeal to a range of students and practitioners across a diverse range of settings spanning health, education and social care. Not all readers will be professionally qualified, but in either case it will be vital that they experience not only personal support for themselves but also supervision of their practice. We all encounter unexpected events and situations in our work with families, and it is essential and ethical that more senior colleagues should be available to consult and advise.

This pendulum swing away from a 'deficiency' model towards a 'strengths' model, both for families and for ourselves, is extremely welcome. It does not mean that we overlook danger signals, but as we shall see when discussing the Signs of Safety approach to child protection (Government of Western Australia 2011) which has now reached the UK, we can acknowledge what is working well for families, at the same time making it clear what further steps need to be taken to protect their child. Such an approach, practised in the context of respecting and supportive relationships, is entirely in line with a focus on strengths.

In a major review of the Signs of Safety approach, commissioned by the National Society for the Prevention of Cruelty to Children (NSPCC), Bunn (2013) introduces this model of practice as follows (p.8):

> Created in Western Australia during the 1990s by Andrew Turnell and Steve Edwards, Signs of Safety is based on the use of Strength Based interview techniques, and draws upon techniques from Solution Focused Brief therapy (SFBT). It aims to work collaboratively and in partnership with families and children to conduct risk assessments and produce action plans for increasing safety, and reducing risk and danger by focusing on strengths, resources and networks that the family have. The model has evolved since the 1990s and has been built on the experiences and feedback of case workers adopting the

Box 9. Key findings from the NSPCC commissioned report on the Signs of Safety model in child protection. (Bunn 2013)

- Practitioners described Signs of Safety as a useful framework for addressing the danger and harm factors in a case and clarifying the concerns, especially with more difficult cases and during periods of crisis. They felt that Signs of Safety helped to identify risk.

- Signs of Safety helped practitioners to be more specific about child protection issues, ensuring they described behaviours and frequencies rather than just saying the child had experienced 'neglect'. This was also thought to help practitioners think of families as individual families, each different, rather than just having a certain 'type' of problem.

- Signs of Safety methods were thought to increase participation, co-operation and the engagement of parents/families.

- Parents liked focusing on strengths and not just problems.

- The approach helped parents to see things from the child's perspective.

- The tools gave younger children a voice and a say.

- Using Signs of Safety means that action and change was more likely to happen.

- There is limited evidence so far on whether Signs of Safety improves outcomes for children.

- Further research is need to evaluate the effectiveness of this model.

- Therapy or psychological assessment. This includes an Education, Health and Care Plan.

It appears then that while the Signs of Safety model of practice has many positive features, sufficient to persuade 'at least 50 jurisdictions in 12 different countries cross Australasia, North America and Europe' to use it, researchers are still urging that more evaluations should be undertaken in order to explore the effectiveness of the model (Bunn, 2013, p.7).

CHAPTER 1

Pregnancy

OVERVIEW

Acknowledging risk factors

Building on protective factors

Engaging with fathers and other family members

Highlighting the strengths of the family

Attending to the parents' wellbeing

Motivational interviewing (MI)

Bonding with the baby during pregnancy

Looking ahead to parenthood

The Family Nurse Partnership

Our aim in this chapter, and indeed in this book, is to acknowledge, highlight and draw attention to the many opportunities which exist for enhancing the wellbeing of young children and their parents, while not ignoring the difficulties which many will encounter. As illustrated in Figure 1.1, there are many challenges and hazards which parents expecting a new baby may have to deal with, but our intention is to acknowledge these while paying much more attention to the ways in which practitioners can actively support parents at this time – and in so doing improve the opportunities for growth and fulfilling development in their children.

Some readers, for example social workers who are seldom routinely involved in the care of women expecting a child, might question why they are invited to become familiar with some of the research relating to pregnancy – a field more often associated with midwives and increasingly with health visitors. There are at least two answers: one, that social workers do often encounter women during their pregnancy when issues of domestic violence arise and a woman with her unborn child needs safeguarding; and two, they often become involved with young mothers-to-be who have become pregnant while still teenagers. It is hoped therefore that the material in this chapter will be seen as important for social workers and their assistants.

ACKNOWLEDGING RISK FACTORS

The primary focus of this book then is on favourable factors which contribute towards wellbeing in childhood and a fulfilled adult life. However, it would be inaccurate and unethical not to acknowledge the potentially damaging influences and events which may prejudice this positive outcome. For example, there is considerable evidence that genetic factors can contribute to the probability of a child having substantial difficulties in later life, including mental health problems and personality difficulties, which may predispose him or her to get into trouble with the law. These difficulties are included at this early stage in the book so that practitioners can familiarise themselves with the evidence emerging from a wide range of disciplines, including research in genetics. Scott (2006), for example, writes:

> ...while the influence of upbringing is still recognised as key, nowadays the unique contribution of the child is better understood. Recent behavioural genetic findings show that some children inherit traits that impair their ability to get on with others and understand their feelings. Three typologies are being increasingly recognised as complicating the picture for some antisocial children, and each is highly heritable. Firstly, severe hyperactivity and inattention can lead to such impulsive responding that the child doesn't have time to reflect before acting – such children are easily seen as emotionally illiterate, and their hyperactivity can be missed due to the salience of the antisocial acts. Then children with Asperger's syndrome or autistic-like traits have difficulty reading emotions and engaging in the basic to-and-fro of day-to-day social encounters, and this... means they easily get frustrated and become aggressive... Finally there is increasing interest in children who seem otherwise intact but display marked callous-unemotional traits. These children seem to understand most emotions, but not to care about distress in others, or to feel much hurt themselves (Viding 2004)... In the extreme, these traits add up

to psychopathy, and in adults this is associated with low activity in the amygdala, the brain region associated with the processing of fear (Blair, Mitchell and Blair 2005).

Notwithstanding this worrying evidence, Scott goes on to emphasise that research is showing that all these groups of children can be helped with specialist parenting programmes. The Maudsley Hospital, in London, is a leading research centre for these programmes; parenting packages, carefully tailored to the characteristics of the children, have been developed in the UK and overseas and have been shown to be effective in rigorous trials (Scott 2006).

The vulnerabilities noted above interact with environmental circumstances. It is now accepted that children who experience the unfolding of their genetically underpinned characteristics in situations of the greatest adversity go on to demonstrate the highest levels of difficulty. There now seems also to be a general consensus that almost all the major difficulties which characterise children arise through a complex interaction of genetic and environmental factors. Clearly, we practitioners have influence over only the environmental ones, but within those constraints there is room for an extensive series of positive interventions to be brought to bear.

To reiterate, abundant evidence shows that socioeconomic factors often play a major role in prejudicing the life of a child and that low income, isolation and poor accommodation are all hazards for mothers and their babies. The evidence concerning the damaging effects on many mothers-to-be of living with low incomes in deprived neighbourhoods is widely confirmed. Dunkel Schetter and Tanner (2012) in a major review have highlighted the effects of homelessness, racism and poverty on pregnant women and the associated low birth weight and premature birth of their babies. Research has focused on several areas of potential difficulty in pregnancy: stress and its impact on the foetus, smoking, prematurity, obstetric difficulties and low weight for dates, as well as pregnancy at a young age. We shall consider each of these fields of research briefly.

Concerning stress in pregnancy, O'Connor and colleagues (2002) are among those who have demonstrated that mothers' marked anxiety in pregnancy can be followed by several undesirable consequences for their children. For example, the children of mothers with high levels of anxiety when they were 18 weeks pregnant did not show any specific consequences, emotionally or behaviourally; however, mothers who were highly anxious at 32 weeks gestation were twice as likely as other mothers to have a child with emotional or behavioural difficulties when they were aged four. More seriously, this team and others have shown that high levels of anxiety in late pregnancy were associated with an increased probability of attention deficit hyperactivity disorder (ADHD) in both boys and girls.

Stress in pregnancy occurs for many reasons: as we saw above, it may arise directly from the woman finding herself pregnant when she was not anticipating this; it may arise from having little money, poor accommodation and alienation from her community; and it may arise from experiencing violence and/or abuse from the father of the child-to-be. We shall consider these circumstances further below.

Smoking during pregnancy, which may well be a habit of stressed mothers as a way of coping with anxiety, poses its own hazards. While different studies have found different levels of risk associated with smoking, the consensus now appears to be that smoking in pregnancy, particularly heavy smoking, interacting with other factors, may be a factor in the children of that pregnancy becoming involved in offending in later life – although the mechanism is as yet unclear (Paradis *et al.* 2011). Similar variability has emerged from a range of studies concerning drinking alcohol during pregnancy: while some authorities suggest that drinking small amounts of alcohol is not dangerous for the foetus, others, including the British Medical Association, recommend ruling out alcohol completely. From attempts to understand the mechanisms involved, it is now known that exposure to nicotine in the case of smoking and to ethanol in the case of drinking alcohol is linked with changes in the baby's neural functioning, which is in turn associated with cognitive deficits and behaviour problems. These contribute towards the likelihood of poor performance in school and thence a slide into truancy and possible offending.

Young mothers, particularly unsupported young mothers, are often coping with many more pressures than are older mothers. While many young parents manage their babies admirably and bring up confident and secure children, others struggle partly through inexperience per se and partly through isolation, loneliness and lack of support. It is notable that when it was decided to introduce the Family Nurse Partnership (FNP) into the UK, following its successful implementation in the United States, its resources and services were directed initially towards new mothers under twenty years of age and their partners. We shall discuss this later in more depth.

Whereas it is now better understood that PND is a major risk factor for both mother and child, the hazards posed by antenatal depression are less well known. In the Western world, up to 20 per cent of women experience antenatal depression, often associated with loneliness, limited social support and the lack of support from a husband or partner. Depression associated with domestic violence is particularly hazardous, as is known from the work of Flach *et al.* (2011), who showed in a study of over 13,000 mothers and their children that antenatal domestic violence was associated with depressive symptoms both before and after the birth of the child, with violence continuing after the birth and with 'future behavioural problems in the child at 42 months'.

BUILDING ON PROTECTIVE FACTORS

Let us turn now to the main focus of this book, namely the positive factors and experiences which offer protection to both parents and child, which can enhance lifelong development and to which we can contribute. We shall consider two specific ones: a confiding relationship for the parents, which may well be linked with a client-centred approach by the helping person; and helping the mother and father with their feelings.

A confiding relationship for parents: the client-centred approach

A supportive relationship with another person in whom she can confide is known to be a powerful protective factor during pregnancy for a young mother-to-be; and the midwife is the natural person with whom such a confiding relationship can be established. The midwifery profession, both in the UK and in Canada and Australia, has undertaken admirable evaluations of different models of practice with mothers-to-be, particularly comparing 'caseload midwifery' with 'team midwifery'. McCourt *et al.* (2006, p.148) clarify:

> Caseload midwifery…[is] a form of practice in which each midwife is responsible for, and provides most of the midwifery care for a caseload of women throughout pregnancy, birth and the early weeks after the baby is born. Midwives' work centres around women rather than being attached to particular clinical locations. They can provide care from a range of locations including hospital, birth centres, women's homes and community settings, according to a woman's needs. In this model the woman and her midwife get to know each other well over the whole maternity experience, building a relationship of trust with each other, sharing information and decision making…

By contrast:

> In the team midwifery model, a small team of midwives provides antenatal, birth and postnatal care for a defined number of women. A team of six midwives may share a caseload of 300–350 women…

These two models of practice are being evaluated in several countries, and each appears to have advantages. In the UK the midwifery profession seems to be working towards a situation where every mother-to-be has a named midwife whom she can anticipate seeing throughout her pregnancy. Many women 'tend to prefer care with a known midwife' and this continuity seems to be particularly important to women in ethnic minority groups (McCourt and Pearce 2000). Time and available resources will show whether this highly desirable arrangement can be universally implemented.

Whether you are a counsellor, a midwife, health visitor, a social worker or a trained volunteer, you will know a good deal about making relationships with a wide range of people. If you are visiting someone at home or meeting them at the health centre, your appreciative, focused attention is likely to make the meeting one which calms and reassures the mother-to-be. Here the work of Carl Rogers, a psychologist, can help us. Rogers (1951) highlighted the necessity of offering 'unconditional positive regard' at all times to those whom he encountered: that is, conveying courtesy and respect to his clients, regardless of their circumstances or how they treated him. There is evidence that those who experienced this courtesy found it profoundly reassuring and beneficial; it paved the way, over time, for a confiding relationship and for the development of trust. Indeed, the results from this study underpinned the development of a new therapeutic approach:

client-centred therapy. Only a few years later an even stronger body of evidence concerning the beneficial contribution to be made to therapy via the person of the counsellor became available. Charles Truax and Robert Carkhuff, already mentioned, published their seminal book, *Towards Effective Counselling and Psychotherapy* in 1967. They pointed out that the evidence available at that time indicated that:

> ...average counselling and psychotherapy is ineffective, but some is indeed effective. (p.5)

These researchers went on examining literally thousands of research studies to establish the characteristics of situations where clients reported that they had been helped and distinguishing them from those where clients reported that they had not been helped. Their findings were that situations concerning the former were not those where the therapist had had a specific theoretical stance, for example psychoanalytic or behavioural, but rather that these clients:

> ...all stressed the importance of the therapist's ability to provide a nonthreatening, trusting, safe or secure atmosphere by his acceptance, nonpossessive warmth, unconditional positive regard or love. Finally, virtually all theories of psychotherapy emphasize that for the therapist to be helpful he must be accurately empathic, be 'with' the client, be understanding, or grasp the patient's meaning. (p.25)

Truax and Carkhuff went on to describe these three sets of characteristics as *accurate empathy*, *nonpossessive warmth* and *genuineness*.

More recently, Asay and Lambert (1999) undertook an extensive analysis of the particular components of effective counselling and psychotherapy and in reporting their work, Fall, Miner Holden and Marquis (2004) noted:

- Forty per cent of positive outcomes in psychotherapy can be attributed to factors essentially out of the counsellor's hands. These include client factors such as the severity and chronicity of the client's problem; the client's level of motivation to change; the client's capacity to relate to other people; the client's ego strength...; the quality of the client's social support system and the client's ability and motivation to access and use self-help and community resources.

- Fifteen per cent of positive outcomes can be attributed to the client's expectation of improvement.

- Thirty per cent of beneficial helpful outcomes can be attributed to the therapeutic relationship.

Or, as we might describe it in this context, the helping relationship. Thirty per cent is a very high figure indeed and one which alerts us to the power for good which we, as people who are hoping to help, may bring to a situation – as well as to the responsibility which we carry for seeing that that potential for good is used well.

In discussing this, Fall *et al.* (2004) confirm: 'It is the counselor's responsibility to establish and maintain, and consistently communicate, acceptance of, warmth toward, and empathy for the client.' They continue:

- Fifteen per cent of positive outcomes can be attributed specifically to the techniques which the therapist uses.

These might include strategies peculiar to a specific theoretical approach, such as keeping a diary or the practice of relaxation.

Now, in considering the ways in which practitioners might develop professional or principled relationships with parents-to-be, we are not talking about therapy, psychotherapy or indeed counselling, but about positive and constructive interactions between professional or lay helpers and parents, either as individuals or with families. So I must ask here whether there is, or should be, any substantial difference between the effective counsellors' ways of relating with their clients and the ways in which helpful health visitors, social workers, mentors, family aides or indeed volunteers relate to those they work with. It is a key principle of the work of health professionals that midwives and health visitors, speech and language therapists, physiotherapists and indeed all such professionals, should offer *accurate empathy, warmth* and *respect* as core features of their attentiveness to their clients. Such ways of relating with people are, or should be, core principles of our professional or lay interactions.

Why are these characteristics so important?

It may be surprising to appreciate that a main reason for the impact of these helper characteristics is grounded in physiology rather than in psychology. Any person who is under stress, even for a common activity such as visiting the dentist, knows that this event is commonly, although not always, very anxiety-provoking. In these circumstances this anxiety is experienced as activity in the hypothalamic-pituitary-adrenal (HPA) system, which leads to increased heart rate, a dry mouth, a churning stomach and sometimes difficulty in breathing, accompanied by sensations of threat. In some contexts, this constellation of experiences will be known as the 'fight-flight-freeze' phenomenon, which in evolutionary times prepared our ancestors to fight and resist a threat forcefully or, if it seemed too powerful, to run away; a third possible response is to stand stock still, every sense alert to an impending threat. If this last response is seen in children who may have been abused it is sometimes known as 'frozen awareness', since the child is too young to resist, has nowhere to flee to and so can only wait, in fear, watching from which direction or from whom the next assault may come. Indeed, the mother or parents whom you are visiting may be experiencing very similar sensations as they wait to meet you, a stranger about whom they know nothing, but someone who probably has power over them and their family.

It will be apparent that encountering someone, be it therapist, counsellor, health visitor or home visiting volunteer, who shows warmth, respect and friendliness will be reassuring to the parents-to-be. Their anxiety levels associated with the prospect of meeting a stranger, who may or may not be a welcome visitor, are likely to reduce and indeed are likely to decrease further when the visitor empathises with them concerning their circumstances – rather than, for example, giving minimal information about themselves and glancing round the room for signs of order or disorder! If these characteristics of friendliness, respect and empathy can be maintained throughout the period of the relationship they are likely to contribute to a positive and constructive encounter between all the participants.

Helping the mother and father with their feelings

We shall not assume that the particular mother whom we are meeting feels happiness about or even acceptance of the impending birth of her child. While a great many parents will be joyful about the pregnancy, a great many others may feel dismayed, desperate, fearful of or hostile to the new life within them. Open statements, such as 'So you're expecting a baby…', as distinct from closed questions, 'How do you feel about being pregnant?' are more likely to enable mothers and fathers gradually to reveal their true feelings. Verbal and non-verbal replies may be contradictory – in which case it is the non-verbal ones which are likely to be the more accurate. Even an apparently positive response delivered in a monotone may well belie the actual feelings involved. The point at issue here is that as the visitor gets to know the mother she will be helping the mother more by enabling her to acknowledge her ambivalence or hostility, rather than by expecting her to be pleased in the conventional ways expected by many cultures. Too ready a response by the practitioner such as, 'Oh, you'll soon get used to the idea' or, 'Count your blessings: many women would love to be expecting a child', will close down the *opportunity to confide* known to be so valuable to people in distress. Acknowledging ambivalent feelings at the present time does not confirm them as fixed and final: rather it opens the way to the possibility of changed feelings on a later occasion. Mothers and fathers may need the opportunity to talk separately if it appears that they feel differently about the pregnancy.

Many visits to new mothers-to-be are likely to include a focus on practical matters such as the expected date of delivery and on which tests and checks the mother has already had. There will probably be discussion of where the birth is to take place – home, hospital or special unit – and on who will be present at the birth to support the mother. Some mothers will have been in touch with midwifery services as soon as they knew they were pregnant; others will come late to those services, either through fear or simple ignorance of what help and reassurance midwives and their assistants can offer. We may hope that these meetings will be reassuring and informative to new mothers-to-be, but this will not always be the case.

Midwives and other professionals too will often encounter women who are deeply ambivalent about their pregnancy, who are reluctant to see it to full term, or who are under pressure from a partner or family to undergo a termination. In these circumstances the woman will be coping with high levels of stress as she tries to understand her new circumstances and their implications for herself, her partner, her family and the developing baby within her. The midwife is one of those with the responsibility for enabling the woman to explore, in the light of all the medical and social circumstances affecting her, what courses of action are open to her. Her active listening will be the more helpful and calming if she conveys respect, warmth and empathy. Helpers who are not professionally qualified will be likely to refer the person concerned to agencies more equipped to explore the implications of the pregnancy with the woman concerned.

Assuming that the pregnancy is going ahead, a main contribution which a professional or well-informed friend can offer is to make regular contact with the mother-to-be. It may well be impossible to visit regularly or frequently, but phone contact may be possible, so enabling the woman to speak freely of her difficulties, her continuing uncertainty about a possible termination or her fears about the response of her partner to her circumstances. If we can offer a confidential listening ear and be available to listen for as long as is possible then we shall be doing much to reduce the stress level of the woman concerned. As we do so, our active listening can convey those very ways of relating identified above: empathy, warmth and unconditional positive regard (see Table 1.1).

Table 1.1 Sympathetic and empathic responses to a worried teenager

Pregnant mum-to-be	Sympathetic response	Empathic response
I wasn't expecting to get pregnant...	You poor thing... What are you going to do?	Finding you're pregnant is a bit of a shock to you...
Yes, he said he didn't like condoms, so I thought I'd take a chance...	These men, they're all alike, just thinking of themselves...	You thought it was unlikely you'd get pregnant...
Yes, I'm really scared to tell my mum. She told me not to go with him...	Yes, your mum can be really scary... Poor you!	The thought of telling your mum is really upsetting for you...
I'd like to get rid of the baby. How can I do that?	Yes, I'm not surprised you're wondering that. I'm really sorry for you...	The idea of a termination is quite appealing to you...
But part of me would like to keep it...	You sound really mixed up... You need to sort out what you want...	You're not sure what you feel about this baby...
Oh dear, I don't know what to do...and I'm already three months gone.	You poor thing... You'd better make your mind up quickly...	You wish you had more time to decide what you really want to do...

It may be that the mother-to-be will allow us, or even ask us, to talk with other important people in her life: her husband or boyfriend, her mother, her father, her sister or her grandparents. Demonstrating an understanding that the pregnancy may be seen very differently by each of these family members and friends may be difficult, but listening to and acknowledging the range of sometimes intense feelings involved can act as a kind of 'pressure valve' and help reduce the strength of opinion being brought to bear upon the young mother-to-be. If we can empathise with family members' feelings, but without endorsing them, we may win their confidence in taking forward whatever decisions have to be made. At this early stage we should avoid premature problem solving but demonstrate rather that we can be trusted with confidential views or information. As we have seen, confiding in a trustworthy friend or reliable confidante has the effect of reducing stress, diminishing anxiety and opening the way to clearer thinking and decision making.

ENGAGING WITH FATHERS AND OTHER FAMILY MEMBERS

Because of the abundant evidence of the positive impact which the support of the father of a child can offer it may be fitting, according to our role, either professional or lay, to explore with the mother-to-be her feelings and attitudes towards the father of the baby. While some mothers have close and supportive relationships with their husbands or partners, others will be ambivalent, especially if the father is none too pleased to find that his partner is pregnant. Some women will want nothing to do with him; others would like his involvement but do not know how to get it. Yet others will still be wondering about the possibility of a termination. Here again the role of a supportive professional or skilled friend is to offer active listening: enabling the mother to explore her feelings and deepest wishes.

Many more fathers are willing to become involved in caring for their children these days than was so as recently as 20 years ago, and this is associated with better cognitive and emotional development in their children (Redshaw and Henderson 2013). In a study of 4616 women in England, more than 80 per cent of fathers were 'pleased' or 'overjoyed' that their partner was pregnant and almost all were present for ultrasound examinations and for the birth. This greater involvement by fathers was associated with several advantages to the baby, including increased levels of breastfeeding. However, these researchers report that 'women in some sociodemographic groups may be less supported by their partner and more reliant on staff...'

A recent Swedish study has described how both expectant mothers and fathers value the primarily medical care which mothers are offered in that country but fathers reported often feeling 'invisible'. Both mothers and fathers would have welcomed more opportunities to meet other parents-to-be in group settings (Widarsson et al. 2012). A further qualitative study by this team (Widarsson et al. 2015) reports fathers' efforts to be involved in their partner's pregnancy as 'paddling upstream': themes such as trying to participate, trying to be understanding, trying to learn, trying to be a calming influence and trying to find a balanced life all emerged as key features of what these fathers-to-be were seeking to achieve. The researchers report: 'Both expectant mothers and fathers wanted the father to be more involved in the pregnancy.

Although fathers attempted different strategies, they did not always perceive what was expected of them and encountered many barriers as they tried to navigate through this unique experience. The best support for the father was the mother.' It may well be that we can follow the lead of Swedish health care professionals in trying both to engage fathers more fully in their partners' pregnancy and also to develop both individual and group strategies for doing so.

Many fathers, young and older, are in great need of a concerned and dispassionate person to talk to, to help them acknowledge the stress and ambivalence they feel on learning that their partner is pregnant. One recent, albeit small, study by Wilkes, Mannix and Jackson (2012) with adolescent and young adult expectant fathers where the pregnancy of their partners was unplanned is a major contribution to this field. The researchers report that 'impending fatherhood presented these young men with mixed emotions and many challenges. The pregnancies were all unplanned and though participants were all willing to face the responsibilities associated with fatherhood, they also reported feeling ill-prepared for the challenges that lay ahead. Impending fatherhood has caused the young men to reflect on the quality of fathering they had received themselves...' Wilkes *et al.* recommend that prenatal classes should include specific sessions for prospective fathers and provide opportunities to assist young men to discuss their thoughts and concerns about impending fatherhood.

Without support the danger is that young fathers may be inclined to deny the reality of the situation in which they find themselves, and to leave the mother-to-be to fend for herself. Here the availability of a male midwife, one of some 170 in the UK, could have a greatly beneficial impact on the wellbeing both of the young father and of the woman and her baby. Young men are likely to feel more comfortable talking to a man, be he midwife, social worker, health visitor or youth worker, in such circumstances and words of empathy and appreciation offered to an extremely stressed young dad may be what are needed for him to keep in touch with and provide support to his partner or girlfriend. Critical comments, such as, 'Now see the trouble you have caused. What are you going to do about it!?', may drive that young man to abandon his partner – particularly if the criticism is frequently repeated; but an empathic response, acknowledging the young man's confusion and ambivalence, can help towards a sensitive discussion of possible courses of action.

In the same way, and if the young woman agrees, it may be fitting for the worker to encourage her to be in touch with members of her family, perhaps a sister, her parents, a grandparent or a more distant relative. In some cases the woman may agree to the practitioner contacting that relative. Many young women, having had an argument with their parents, have decided to move out from the family home and are struggling to cope alone, or with minimal family contact. If this arrangement is working and the mother-to-be is content with it, there may be little to be done; but if she is half wishing that she were still in contact with her mum, or with a sister, then with permission, sensitive liaison with those family members could be invaluable to all concerned.

HIGHLIGHTING THE STRENGTHS OF THE FAMILY

A very important study, again drawn from research in counselling, concerns the great value of the practitioner's deliberately adopting an actively encouraging and positive tone in their interactions with clients or those they are seeking to help. Fluckiger and Grosse Holtforth (2008) in a seminal study have reported that when trainee psychotherapists spent five minutes before each of the first five meetings with a client talking with a colleague about their client's strengths and how successfully they had reminded clients of those strengths, this practice had had a marked positive effect on relationships *and outcomes* (my italics). These results were not found in a control group where counsellors did not actively draw attention to the clients' strengths. Indeed, in the last few years the importance of an early positive focus on the strengths of the client (as distinct from a focus on problems) has been repeatedly demonstrated as eliciting optimism, hope and motivation among clients.

We are not talking here of premature or empty praise, but of clients' identifiable strengths as they become evident in the course of early discussion. Many parents do not recognise their past achievements or future potential and until they are elicited from them by sensitive listening or gentle enquiry they may well be discounted. I recall my own amazement when I enquired of a young mother whom I was visiting whether there was anything in her life before she became a mum which gave her pleasure to think about? 'Well,' she said tentatively, 'I used to row for England…' I was dumbfounded. Here was a young mother, deeply depressed by her current life circumstances, whose previous achievements she totally disregarded under the pressure of coping with her rather naughty and disruptive two-year-old. It was my job not to overplay that achievement, but to draw from all the life experience, commitment and motivation which that success must have required of her, to help revive her energies in caring for her little dynamo of a toddler. Together, we were able to do this.

Practitioners who follow a solution-focused model of practice typically deliberately pay a compliment to the people early in the contact with a person whom they are trying to help. Students being trained within this approach are taught early in their contact with a client to identify some praiseworthy aspect of his or her life or behaviour in order to 'reward' the person in some way. This might be the efforts which the person has made to deal with a very demanding situation, or the concern which she or he shows for the wellbeing of family members. The appreciation by the practitioner is offered explicitly, openly and sincerely. Physiologically, the experience of 'reward', in this case appreciation, involves key brain systems including the mesolimbic and mesocortical pathways. Activity in these systems tends to counter anxiety and is likely to reassure the parent that the visitor is positive, appreciative and not bent on finding fault.

ATTENDING TO THE PARENTS' WELLBEING

Even if the helper is not a qualified health professional, it would be entirely appropriate for him or her actively to attend to the physical wellbeing of the parents and their baby. This might include gently exploring with the mother how she is feeling in herself, whether she has support from family members or friends, whether she is in touch with her midwife – so as to receive available dietary supplements and other benefits, to book necessary scans and to have her own health monitored. There should be similar support for the father as well.

If the mum-to-be is frightened of meeting the midwife, and her own mother or sister is not available to accompany her, then the helper can offer to go along as a 'buddy'; having a trusted person to take this role can be a great reassurance to the mother once the relationship has 'gelled'. The buddy can, as appropriate, go with the mother to her scans and to the appointments with the midwife. She can make notes about suggestions made by the midwife for clarification and discussion later. If the first language of the mother is not English, then the buddy can liaise with the interpreter and clarify that advice from the midwife is well understood by the mother. In such circumstances the role of the buddy may be absolutely critical.

Some mothers will already be in touch with their midwife but others will not, and there may well be implications of this. Generally, practitioners can make it clear that the conversations between themselves and the parents are confidential, with the proviso that should matters arise which raise concerns about the wellbeing of the baby to be born, then the practitioner is duty bound to report this to the authorities.

If either parent seems to want to explore the possibility of a termination of the pregnancy, then the worker needs to acknowledge their concern; but then, according to her professional role and responsibilities, she should seek the guidance of her supervisor as a matter of urgency.

Although family nurses attached to the FNP initiative, which we shall discuss in greater detail later in this chapter, typically meet with mothers about fortnightly to monitor the mother's health and the progress and outcomes of scans, it is rare that this frequency of contact will be possible for regular midwives or lay practitioners. Nonetheless, it can be reassuring to mothers to know that their wellbeing is being monitored by experienced workers, who can gently raise topics such as smoking and/or the taking of drugs or alcohol during the pregnancy.

Support for families with English as a second language

The task of communicating across language and cultural barriers becomes ever more challenging. Mares, Henley and Baxter (1985), working in the health care field, have suggested five practical ways in which practitioners can communicate more effectively with people who speak little English or who speak English as a second language (Box 1.1).

Box 1.1 Communicating across language and cultural barriers (after Mares *et al.* 1985)

1 Reduce stress/arousal

- Allow more time than you would for an English-speaking client.
- Give plenty of non-verbal reassurance, by smiling and nodding – if this is in line with cultural convention.
- Get the person's name right and pronounce it correctly.
- Try to ensure that the person meets with the same worker throughout.
- Write down any important points clearly and simply for the person to take away.
- Try to convey something about what will happen next.

2 Simplify your English

- Plan beforehand what you want to communicate to the person.
- Be clear what are the essential points to be conveyed.
- Speak clearly but do not raise your voice.
- Repeat when you think you have not been understood; don't change the words.
- Use words the person is likely to know.
- Don't use slang idioms: for example, 'red tape' or 'spend a penny'.
- Use the simple forms of verbs, active not passive: for example, 'I shall send you a letter', not, 'You'll be sent a letter'.
- Stay with one topic at a time.

3 Check back clearly

- Develop a regular pattern of checking that what you have said so far has been understood.
- Try not to ask, 'Do you understand?' You are almost bound to get 'Yes' as an answer.
- If possible, ask the person to explain back to you what you have suggested.

4 Points to think about when using an interpreter

- The interpreter is to be regarded as an interpreter, not an intermediary.
- Try to give two or three times as much time when working with an interpreter.
- Sit facing the person rather than the interpreter.
- Check that the person and interpreter speak the same language/dialect.
- Appreciate how difficult it may be for newcomers to the country to say 'No' to a person in authority.
- Is there any reason why the person may be embarrassed by the interpreter?
- Might the person find it difficult to tell you things because of the interpreter?
- Is there any reason why the interpreter might be reluctant to interpret things that the person says?
- Does the interpreter understand the purpose of the session and the questions?

5 Learn a few words in the client's language

- Words of greeting or farewell can convey courtesy and respect.

When meeting with people from different cultural or language groups, it is appropriate to acknowledge that you have limited knowledge of these groups, and ask them to tell you if there are important practices which you should respect when meeting them or family members. Ask too that they inform you if you unintentionally neglect or fail to give sufficient attention to a particular issue.

It will be important, when meeting a woman who is pregnant, or members of her family, to know in advance any cultural or dietary practices which need to be attended to – whether it is to be a home or hospital birth. The presence of fathers or other males in the delivery room will be an important matter for discussion, usually of course with the midwife, but this may arise with a volunteer helper also. The issues need to be clarified very well in advance of delivery.

MOTIVATIONAL INTERVIEWING (MI)

It will be apparent to both professionals and lay practitioners who work with parents that there are real risks to the foetus if mothers-to-be and, to a lesser extent, fathers-to-be, smoke or take banned substances while the mother is pregnant. It is becoming common knowledge that these activities are actively dangerous to the developing baby, both in terms of his or her development while in the womb, and in terms of wellbeing after birth. So general practitioners (GPs) and midwives are likely all to be attempting to dissuade parents from smoking, drinking and using drugs, often with discouraging outcomes.

So we turn now to MI, a skill distinguished and propounded by Rollnick, Miller and Butler (2008) in their seminal book, *Motivational Interviewing in Health Care*. This was a development from earlier books on the same theme. It acknowledges that many people who enter the helping professions and take up their helping roles see others taking misguided steps in the course of their lives; these steps are likely ultimately to have negative, if not dangerous, effects for themselves, for others who care about them and for those for whom they are responsible – particularly their children. These misguided steps during pregnancy include smoking tobacco, drinking alcohol and ingesting drugs.

However, the authors point out that the natural response of most of us when we are advised not to pursue an enjoyable activity, especially if it reduces stress, is to resist that advice, and the more strongly the advice is offered, the stronger may be our opposition to it. The authors have therefore distinguished four key principles for those of us bent upon proffering good advice, encapsulated in the mnemonic RULE, as set out in Table 1.2.

Table 1.2 Motivational interviewing: guidelines for working with people in health care settings (Rollnik *et al.* 2008)

Key letter	Guidance
R Resist the righting impulse	We should check our own impulse to correct the behaviour of the person we seek to help. While our motives are sound, attempting to confront the person in order to correct behaviour is likely to be counter-productive.
U Understand the person's motivations	As Rollnick *et al.* phrase it: 'If your consultation time is limited, you are better off asking patients why they would want to make a change and how they might do it rather than telling them that they should'.
L Listen to the patient	We have already referred to the value, indeed the necessity, of enabling the other person to talk freely and in confidence about their circumstances, while we attempt to listen with respect and empathy. Such sensitive attention is intrinsically helpful as it allows anxieties to be voiced, stressors to be identified and the person's overall level of tension to diminish. It enables us, as listeners, to become alert to the half-expressed fear, the barely-voiced anger as well as the longed-for life change.
E Empower the person	This principle concerns how we can help people explore the possibilities of how to enhance their own health or situation. The worker's role is to encourage those explorations of why they might want to make a change and how they might achieve it and then to support their early tentative steps towards that change.

Consider the circumstances of a young mother-to-be, in the early stage of pregnancy, who is smoking heavily but who knows that this is unwise. If we raise the issue too suddenly or too sharply she is likely to 'back off': she may not want to discuss her smoking or even mention it. She may claim to have stopped smoking or be unwilling to meet us at all. It would probably be unprofessional, or at least inappropriate, to avoid talking about the issue altogether, but if the young mum does not refer to it, how should we proceed? Smoking will almost certainly feature on the documentation which midwives are required to complete, but a non-judgemental approach is likely to achieve a greater readiness to confide than a more critical one.

We explore in Table 1.3 some of the pros and cons of smoking which mothers-to-be or their partners who smoke are likely to suggest.

Table 1.3 Pros and cons of smoking suggested by parents	
Advantages of smoking	**Disadvantages of smoking**
It takes away the stress – relaxes you	Expense
Something to do with your hands	It makes your breath smell
You're in with the crowd	Some people avoid you
Easy to carry around	Might get cancer
Smoking doesn't make you drunk	Might harm the baby

BONDING WITH THE BABY DURING PREGNANCY

There is to date only a modest amount of research literature on this topic – for example, the work of Alhusen (2008) – but this has been sufficient to show that maternal and paternal bonding with the foetus is commonly reported and that it is a healthy phenomenon. Parents often tell midwives that they talk and sing to their unborn child and that this gives them an increasing sense of familiarity with him or her – one which comes to full fruition only when the baby is born. A study by Lee and Kisilevsky (2014) was devised in which both mothers and fathers read to the foetus every day for seven days. When the babies were born, recordings were played to the babies and their heart rates and head turnings were carefully recorded. The evidence showed that foetuses responded to both parents' voices, but they preferred their mother's voice after birth. This area of research continues to expand. It seems, however, that family visitors can usefully encourage parents-to-be to talk and sing to their babies, while being aware that there might be dangers in arriving at fully developed images of what the baby might look like and what his or her personality might be.

LOOKING AHEAD TO PARENTHOOD

While, typically, the preoccupations of parents during pregnancy centre upon the next few months and the birth of their baby, it may well be possible to help parents to discuss the care of the baby in the earliest months of life. Here is an area where the helper should try to involve both parents in the discussions: the evidence is that if it can be taken for granted that there is a clear role for both parents in caring for the baby, this will be beneficial to both the baby and the parents themselves (Ramchandani *et al.* 2013).

Preparing to look after the baby

Unless the mother is fortunate enough to have had access to small nieces and nephews or other small babies and children she may be fearful of the responsibilities of caring for a tiny baby. In my own case, I had not even held a baby before my own was born and I was utterly unprepared for the stress and fatigue which accompanied her early days. Fortunately, a helpful nurse had shown me how to hold the baby to feed her, how to bath her and how to change nappies, and if it is the case that mothers-to-be are as inexperienced as I, these are activities which can be practised during the pregnancy with a soft cuddly doll.

At the least, it will be fitting tactfully to explore the parents' intentions about feeding the baby. There is abundant evidence that breastfeeding is highly desirable for the infant, but as discussed above, to over-emphasise this will be counter-productive. We shall return to breastfeeding in the next chapter, but it is probably wise to leave the subject open at this stage. This is the time when, it is to be hoped, the parents are assembling a good supply of nappies, creams and baby garments – in several sizes. It is likely that they will be given an assortment of vests, baby-grows and other clothing, but if not the helper can ask among her own friends and acquaintances.

The parents' plans for the future can, over the course of time, be explored. In the early months, what sources of active help will be available? Will the father take paternity leave? How does he feel about this? Where will the baby sleep? Do the parents plan to make use of nursery care?

Ideally, the visitor can help the mother to think beyond the arrival of the baby, although of course the mother's whole focus is on the impending birth, both physiologically and emotionally. I remember how I took a pile of books into hospital with me, anticipating following up my interest in history. I did not read, or even look into, a single one of them: Nature took over and my hormones ensured that my full attention, for days, weeks, months and years, was focused on my baby girl.

Yet gradually other events did become important again: I did not go back to work, but we planned to go, and eventually went, to India where my husband taught, and so a certain amount of planning in managing the events of our lives had to take place. Similarly, if the helper can enable the mother to make an outline plan for the baby's and her own health, they will have worked together at least on the plan of a plan (Box 1.2).

Box 1.2 Topics to help parents plan a plan

1. After the birth of the baby, what are the plans of the mother and father?

2. Do they plan to return to work?

3. If so, who will care for the baby?

4. If the baby is to go to a nursery, which one?

5. What about the costs/travel costs of the nursery place?

6. Who will take the baby to and from the nursery?

7. What support can the father or other relative give?

8. What work may be available for the mother?

9. Etc., etc.

THE FAMILY NURSE PARTNERSHIP

The FNP, referred to briefly above, is an evidence-based initiative developed in the United States and now available in many cities in the UK; it focuses on the prevention of difficulties for parents and child by offering them support and guidance from pregnancy onwards. The programme is typically offered to first-time young mothers and the same practitioner, often a midwife or health visitor, works with the family from early pregnancy until the child is aged two years.

The FNP is focused on young mothers aged less than 20 years and their first babies. It is one of the most successful of the many packages of care which have been brought to the UK because of the rigour of the evaluations which have been undertaken in the USA. The team of Olds *et al.* (1998) demonstrated that the children of young mothers who took part in the programme enjoyed better health, better achievement in school, and fewer problems in childhood and in adolescence, while the mothers too benefited significantly. Participation is voluntary and, once accepted onto the programme, the mother receives fortnightly visits from a family nurse – in the UK typically a health visitor – during the nine months of the pregnancy and then, after the birth, monthly until the child is two years old (Box 1.3). The visiting nurse or health visitor receives extensive training beyond the professional qualifications she already holds, and so, using these skills and her own sensitivity and empathy, she works to develop a supportive and caring relationship with the young mother (Eckenrode *et al.* 2010).

We have already considered some of the domains which the family nurse addresses in her regular meetings with the mothers: building supportive relationships with the father of the baby and, it is hoped, with the young woman's family network. She will tactfully discuss the health of the mother and any patterns of smoking or drug use together with her nutrition and exercise, her accommodation and the support she receives from local community resources. In addition, however, the family nurse works with the young woman to consider her life course, her educational record and any plans she has for resuming study or training after the birth of the baby; and of course she will focus on the baby's wellbeing, the mother's understanding of the changes taking place in her body and the needs of the baby after birth. Throughout, the aim is to empower the mother, to prepare her for the impending changes to her body and life, to enhance her health and to enable her to enjoy her pregnancy by preparing as fully as possible for the new arrival.

Box 1.3 Domains addressed by Family Nurse Partnership practitioners

- *Personal health.* The family nurse supports the mother's personal health, including her nutrition and exercise, her use of drugs and alcohol and maintaining mental wellbeing.
- *Environmental health.* The family nurse makes sure that the mother and child have adequate housing and support from their community.
- *Life course development.* The mother and family nurse work in partnership to identify relevant goals for the mother. These goals typically involve plans for the mother to complete her education, find a job and postpone the birth of a second child.
- *Maternal role.* The family nurse works with the mother to help her develop the knowledge and skills to confidently support the health and development of her child.
- *Friends and family.* The family nurse works with the mother to understand and manage her relationships with others (including her own parents and the baby's father) so that they are supportive of the mother's and child's needs.
- *Health and human services.* The family nurse makes sure that the mother is receiving the optimal amount of support from community resources to meet her family's needs.
- *Pregnancy advice.* The family nurse makes sure that the mother is attending her pregnancy appointments and that she is prepared for the birth of her child.

CHAPTER 2

Birth and the First Year of Life

OVERVIEW

- Acknowledging risk factors
- Building on protective factors
- Supporting new parents: helping to reduce stress
- Supporting breastfeeding
- Getting sleeping patterns off to a good start
- Supporting recovery from PND
- Using ideas from CBT
- Supporting parent-to-infant bonding
- Encouraging father involvement
- Encouraging baby massage
- Supporting the beginnings of infant-to-parent attachment
- Encouraging play and early communication
- Support for parents or infants with learning disabilities

The birth of a new baby is usually a time of great happiness and one accompanied by rejoicing in the extended family: visitors come to see the new arrival, presents are brought, names are discussed and cultural ceremonies associated with birth are arranged. However, giving birth and the events that surround it can also be a time of huge stress, not only for the mother but also for the father and the whole family. Many parents who have given birth will know that this process, however 'natural', can make enormous demands, physiological, physical, emotional and practical, on the parents, especially the mother, and on the baby too as he or she struggles to adjust to life beyond the womb.

In this chapter, as before, we shall focus briefly on risk factors for the child before going on to examine much more fully what support can be offered by both professionals and family, friends and accredited volunteers.

ACKNOWLEDGING RISK FACTORS

The birth itself and its circumstances are times of potential hazard for both the present and the future of the child. As my colleague Vivette Glover and I wrote in an earlier publication: 'There is substantial evidence that premature birth and obstetric difficulties pose substantial risks to the developing child. Low birth weight is widely recognised as a risk factor for a range of subsequent difficulties... An infant with low birth weight is at increased risk of neurological impairment and of experiencing more cognitive difficulties than a child with higher birth weight' (Sutton and Glover 2004).

If such difficulties occur in the context of serious socioeconomic adversity for the family, the levels of risk for the child can begin to accumulate. However, as we shall see, supportive intervention can to some extent offset these risks.

So, first, let us acknowledge the impact of social deprivation and disadvantage on mothers and babies. Poor mothers-to-be are more likely to have low-quality accommodation and to be isolated – circumstances which can lead to depression and to chronic levels of anxiety (Latendresse 2009). These emotions will be intensified by domestic violence or abuse, which has particularly damaging effects. PND poses hazards for many stages of the developing infant's life. For example, a depressed mother may be literally unable to offer the smiling, loving patterns of interaction which elicit her baby's response to her and to other caregivers (Tronick and Reck 2009). If all goes well, however, the mother's interaction with her child will underpin not only the processes of bonding (mother to infant) but also those of attachment (infant to mother/father and other caregivers).

Yet bonding with the child is not a willed choice on the part of a mother or father. It is now known that the level of the hormone oxytocin in pregnant women *predicts* the mother–child bond as displayed by the talk, touch, gaze and expressed emotion of the mother (Feldman *et al.* 2007). Happily, these developments usually occur spontaneously, triggered by the intense hormonal processes which accompany childbirth and leading to the development of intimate bonding relationships between mother, and in due course, father, and child. It remains the case, however, that while many mothers report feelings of intense closeness and love for their baby immediately upon birth, and experience immediate bonding, others report only the gradual development of a sense of closeness and protectiveness – while yet others never achieve the level of intimacy known to be such a powerful protective factor in child development.

A further risk to young children's development is the want of an enjoyable and stimulating environment, provided ideally by loving and encouraging parents and family. Highly stressed mothers do not typically have time, interest or resources to enjoy talking to, playing with and interacting with their new babies, yet the research is clear: this is the very time when those activities are most needed and have the most positive impacts on the developing young child.

It is tempting for parents stressed by multiple demands, with a shortage of family or other human support and desperate for a bit of time to themselves or for household chores, to make use of the 'electronic babysitter', the television. Indeed, in the United States currently 90 per cent of children younger than two years watch some form of electronic media and by three years almost one third of children have a television in their bedrooms. However, this practice cannot be recommended. For example, a Dutch study (Verlinden *et al.* 2012) focusing on slightly older children, aged 18 months, showed that 'high television exposure increases the risk of the incidence and the persistence of externalizing problems in preschool children.' Indeed, the American Academy of Pediatrics (2013) recommends the following practices to parents:

- Discourage screen media exposure to children less than two years of age.
- Limit the total amount of screen time to one to two hours per day.
- Keep the TV set and internet-connected electronic-linked devices out of the child's bedroom.

Rowan, Doan and Cash (2014) have gone further and made recommendations for technology viewing for children from birth to 18 years as shown in Table 2.1.

Using a nationally representative sample, Zimmerman and Christakis (2005) measured the effects on children aged under three years who watched an average of 2.2 hours of television daily, and found modest adverse effects of this on their subsequent cognitive development. They concluded: 'These results suggest that greater adherence to the American Academy of Pediatrics guidelines that children younger than two years not watch television is warranted.' Other effects which were not explored included the number of hours not spent in interacting with other children or adults, hours of sleep lost, and missed opportunities for play with items in the natural world or in the household. The same authorities, in line with the American Academy of Pediatrics, have urged that children, particularly young children, should not have television sets in their bedrooms.

Table 2.1 Technology use: recommended guidelines for children and young people (after Rowan *et al.* 2014)

Developmental age	How much?	Non-violent TV	Hand-held devices	Non-violent video games	Violent video games	Online violent video games or pornography
0–2 years	None	Never	Never	Never	Never	Never
3–5 years	1 hr/day	Yes	Never	Never	Never	Never
6–12 years	2 hrs/day	Yes	Never	Never	Never	Never
13–18 years	2 hrs/day	Yes	Yes	30 mins/day	Never	Never

BUILDING ON PROTECTIVE FACTORS

These are varied and interacting, as shown earlier in Figure I.1. Here we briefly examine some of the main bodies of evidence concerning supportive factors and how helping practitioners can draw upon them for practice.

Drawing on insights from the work of Berry Brazelton

Great efforts are being made in many localities for mothers to meet the health visitor who will be in contact with them as their infant develops before the birth of the baby. For parents, especially first-time mothers, to have met their health visitor, who can build an early relationship and give valuable pre-birth information in conjunction with the midwife, is likely to be a valuable and reassuring contact for all concerned. It is shortage of staff rather than opposition to the principle which is slowing down the arrangement.

The name Berry Brazelton is gradually becoming better known in the UK as his groundbreaking work in the USA, focusing on newborn babies, their readiness for life in the world and their responsiveness to people, is recognised and developed here. Special observers have been trained to introduce parents to, and use with them, the manual The Newborn Behavioral Observations (NBO) System Handbook, included in Understanding Newborn Early Relationships (Nugent, Keefer et al. 2007). This proposed 16 features, including responsiveness to a flashlight, response to sound, muscle tone, crying and soothability, which can all be observed if parents know how, or can learn how, to interpret the baby's key signs and behaviours. However, Nugent *et al.* (2007) insist that it is important that parents understand 'that the NBO is *not* a diagnostic examination designed to identify pathological or atypical signs… Rather, it is [an]…approach designed to describe the infant's behavioural capacities and to join parents in identifying the kinds of caregiving strategies that are best suited to the infant's needs.' For example, while some babies actively enjoy plenty of visual stimulation, others can be easily overwhelmed by too many mobiles or paintings on the sides of cots; the assessor can help parents to distinguish the preferences of the newborn child and to provide resources accordingly.

Parents are typically amazed and delighted to see the individual responsiveness of their new baby and how, under varied circumstances, he or she shows preferences for light, colour and human interaction. They are alerted to the impact of their own behaviour on their baby and become attuned to reading his or her moods or wishes as conveyed through eye movements and facial expressions. Bidmead and Andrews (2004) have summarised the six states distinguished by Brazelton, as shown in Box 2.1.

Box 2.1 Characteristics of infant states:
Nugent (1985), as reported by
Bidmead and Andrews (2004)

State 1 *Deep sleep:* regular breathing, eyes closed, not REM sleep. No spontaneous movements; startles may appear.

State 2 *Light sleep:* irregular breathing, more modulated motor activity. Eyes closed, REM sleep.

State 3 *Semi-alert (drowsy):* baby is semi-alert, with eyes open and/or closed, with variable activity levels.

State 4 *Quiet alert:* baby is looking bright with minimal motor activity.

State 5 *Busy alert:* lots of motor activity with eyes open; fussing may or may not be present.

State 6 *Crying.*

It is likely that the optimal time for parents to interact with their babies is when they are in State 4: Quiet alert. Bidmead and Mackinder (2004 p.473) suggest that, as part of play activities, it is helpful for parents to talk to their baby and comment:

> Talking to a baby and pausing to allow them to make noises or just to mouth in reply, helps them to develop the art of conversation. As the parents pause in expectation of their baby's response, the baby is given an experience of being listened to...

They continue: 'If the parent spends some time playing with their baby, praising them and talking about what is happening around them, making the play more interesting, the baby will concentrate for longer and this will increase their attention span.' Such enhanced ability to concentrate will of course lay down the foundations for the baby to develop communication skills on his or her own account and will in due course prepare them for linguistic abilities and conversation. Practitioners, while not pretending to be formal Brazelton specialists, can also develop abilities to observe tiny, even newborn, babies and to share their insights with parents.

SUPPORTING NEW PARENTS: HELPING TO REDUCE STRESS
A confiding relationship

We saw in Chapter 1, on pregnancy, that abundant research, and specifically the seminal work of Truax and Carkhuff (1967), has shown that a relationship characterised by warmth, empathy and genuineness has a powerfully beneficial impact on people in distress. We saw also that Fall *et al.* (2004), who analysed the impact of different elements of the counselling experience, concluded that thirty per cent of beneficial helpful outcomes can be attributed to the therapeutic relationship. If a therapeutic or supportive relationship carries such potential for good, we should be careful to give it time to flower, to spend time just attending to the new mother and father and showing empathy for the mother's experience of giving birth and for the adjustments which both are having to make to their new circumstances.

A highly experienced and skilled health visitor known to me explained how, following her own traumatic experience of giving birth, she sits down with the mother at the first visit following the birth, and says, 'I wonder what giving birth was like for you.' If the event has been smooth and happy, she moves on to the next topic, but if it has been difficult or dangerous she carefully devotes as much time as she can to listening to the mother's account of her experience and empathising with her as she speaks. For some mothers, this will be their first opportunity of recounting what she *really* felt like both at the time, when labour went on for hours and hours, and more recently when memories of the fear and pain may, or may not, have subsided. In my own case, when I assumed that because I had attended antenatal classes and was looking forward to becoming a mother, giving birth would be a smooth and straightforward event, the shock of the level of pain I experienced and the total unexpectedness of the hours of labour which I underwent made giving birth a very frightening and distressing event.

Exploring financial assistance

Many new parents are desperately short of money, and one of the main ways in which practitioners can support them is by educating themselves about the financial benefits and entitlements for which the parents may be eligible. Although it is probably unwise for practitioners to advise parents themselves, it is obviously sensible for them to know the fundamentals of entitlements. They can encourage parents to get accurate information about their benefits from Job Centre Plus offices or from Citizens Advice Bureau. A wide range of entitlements are available and skilled advice is necessary.

Helping parents develop a routine for themselves – one possible routine.

Box 2.2 A template for a day's routine

- Have a 'To do' list for a given day with no more than five or six items on it.

- Divide the day into three sessions, morning, afternoon, evening, so that a simple routine can be planned for each session – probably with no more than two items listed for each session. For example, 'Feed the baby' and 'Get dressed' may well be real achievements for some exhausted mums, who have found themselves spending all day in their nighties because their babies have been so demanding. But if they have been able to do these tasks, they will have done well, and deserve to be told so: if they haven't, tomorrow is another day.

- Recognise that they are not likely to finish all six tasks, so start each day afresh.

- With babies and young children to care for, achieving the routine of care, for example feed, meal, laundry and bath/ bedtime, is probably quite enough for several weeks.

- Help them to reward themselves with some small treat – a cup of coffee or five minutes with the newspaper – and to praise themselves when they have ticked a goal on the list, for example 'Well done, me!' This is really important.

- Try to let the routine centre round meal times; getting some basic food on the table is a major achievement for weary parents.
- Help them to try to build in a spell of time for themselves and remind them that they need to recharge their batteries. So a bath or a shower, undisturbed, can feel wonderful!
- The helper needs to be a source of praise and encouragement for new parents and to commend each day's achievement, however modest.

Building maternal confidence

Many first-time parents are very low in confidence and need, as we have said, a great deal of sensitive support. If all goes well, this confidence increases with growing familiarity with the baby and with the learning of new skills in discovering how to deal with difficulties and how to enjoy caring for him or her. Often caring for a second child seems much less stressful because many of the situations encountered will not be for the first time and parents bring a wealth of knowledge and experience to looking after this child.

There is often, but not always, a marked increase of confidence during the course of the first year of life and for this reason we have included as Appendix 1 the Maternal Confidence Questionnaire (Dilmore 2004) with 14 questions representing levels of confidence. Inviting a new mother to complete this at, say, three months, six months and one year is likely to show marked changes in confidence over time, but also to highlight areas where particular support may be needed. Among a range of results, Dilmore found that there was a positive correlation between maternal confidence and the size of the mother's support system. Here is where the advantages of having an extended family become apparent: if mother or father have a parent or sister available to take the baby for a walk in the afternoons to enable the breastfeeding mother to catch up on sleep, what a blessing!

SUPPORTING BREASTFEEDING

Innumerable studies have demonstrated the advantages of breastfeeding for both baby and mother. While it is recommended by advisory organisations such as the Department of Health (2011) and the Baby Friendly Initiative (UNICEF 2013) that breastfeeding is ordinarily all that is needed until the baby is six months old, shorter periods are still valuable, particularly if it can be practised for at least three months. In these circumstances, benefits for the baby include less chance of developing eczema, diarrhoea and vomiting and of hospital admission for these conditions, less chance of constipation, and less likelihood of developing obesity and type 2 diabetes in childhood or adulthood.

Equally important is the evidence, gathered via several meta-analyses, that breastfeeding is associated with significantly higher scores for cognitive development than is formula feeding (e.g. Anderson, Johnstone and Remley 1999). Since having low levels of cognitive ability has emerged from abundant research as risk factors for subsequent offending in young people, it is clearly advantageous for mothers to breastfeed their babies, even though the link with cognitive development in their infants is unlikely to seem important when trying to get breastfeeding established!

There are many advantages for the mother who breastfeeds: a lower risk of breast and ovarian cancer and lower levels of hip fractures and osteoporosis in later life – as well as a great saving of money and time. Breastfeeding also leads naturally to the development of a close bond between mother and baby (Turck 2005). Breastfeeding groups have been set up in many Children's Centres with breastfeeding buddies available to help less experienced mothers.

Many mothers, however, are anxious about breastfeeding, often for social reasons, and many teenage mothers are unimpressed by reports of long-term benefits. In working to encourage this age group of mothers to start breastfeeding, Bonyata (2011) suggests the approaches shown in Box 2.3.

Box 2.3 Ways to encourage a teenage
mother to breastfeed (Bonyata 2011)

- Involve a teenage mother who is successfully breastfeeding to act as a model and to give encouragement.

- Emphasise the current advantages of breastfeeding: savings of cost and time.

- Explain that there are advantages to breastfeeding *now*, rather than in the future; for example, the mother will get her weight and figure back much faster if she breastfeeds than if she bottle feeds.

- Explain that breastfeeding will be much better for the baby's health.

- Explain that breastfeeding will be much better for the mother's own health in later years.

GETTING SLEEPING PATTERNS OFF TO A GOOD START

The stresses of giving birth and adjusting to the demands of caring for a new baby can be overwhelming, and this is not the place to go into detailed exploration of issues which are really the province of the health visitor. A key variable in whether the new parents cope or not is likely to be the amount of support, practical and emotional, which they receive during the early months of the baby's life. This support will be all the more crucial if there are already other children in the family. Ideally, of course, this support comes from the extended family and grandparents, sisters and other relatives who can be present to care for the baby and, at the very least, to enable exhausted mothers and fathers to catch up on sleep.

This support needs, of course, to be available throughout the first months and years of life. New parents, who may have grown up in nuclear families, are unlikely to have learned skills of caring for crying, sometimes inconsolable, babies from first-hand experience: it is all so new, overpoweringly new and intensely stressful. Alas, one way to reduce stress is to hit the object of one's frustration and the evidence from a major American study suggests that 'spanking increases with child age. At 9 or 10 months, only 10 per cent of children are spanked. This rises to 15% by 12 months, 25% by 15 months and about 40% by 18 months. By the time children are age 20 months or older, 40% of children are spanked' (MacKenzie *et al.* 2011, 2012). Above all, family workers need to find methods of supporting parents so that they do not spank, or even worse, shake their tiny babies. **Babies must never be shaken.**

If the parents are fortunate enough to be participants in the FNP (Nurse Family partnership in the USA), which was described in Chapter 1, and so receive regular visits from a specially trained health visitor, they may be able to tell her of the pressures and stresses they are coping with. She, in turn, will be able to listen while the parents weep, tell her about their fears and anxieties and, often, offer helpful suggestions. She may speak of baby-soothing tapes for inconsolable infants, or give the telephone number of the CRY-sis organisation[1]:

There are also valuable resources available on YouTube. An appealing production, and one with a helpful and constructive message, includes information such as that babies 'cry more between 4 and 12 weeks but that it usually ends at around 16 weeks'.[2]

I have written elsewhere (Sutton 2006) of some of the ways we can 'come alongside' deeply stressed families. I wrote then that in the context of research into children's sleeping difficulties, Keefe *et al.* (1997) have developed a useful mnemonic, REST, which I reproduce below. The details were developed for social workers and health visitors who might be seen as concerned about child welfare, but the principles are valid for all practitioners trying to help new parents.

---

1   08451 228 669 see also www.cry-sis.org.uk.
2   See *Coping When Your Baby Can't Stop Crying*, www.youtube.com/watch?v=yZkVu19c41I.

Table 2.2 REST: essentials of an approach to help stressed parents (Keefe *et al.* 1997)

Key component	Examples
R Reassurance	That the worker is not seeking to remove the child. That the situation the family is dealing with is not uncommon. That the worker is experienced in dealing with the difficulty in question.
E Empathy	Conveyed by sensitive listening and reflecting feelings with all of the family members for the stresses they are coping with.
S Structure	By using a straightforward approach which makes sense to parents; for example ASPIRE: ASsessment, Planning, Implementation and REview.
T Time out for parents	By trying to arrange respite for parents, for example from community resources or support.

Because shortage of sleep is so stressful for parents, I offer in Box 2.4 the steps suggested by Nikolopoulou and St. James-Roberts (2003) for helping families gradually to assist new babies to sleep through the night.

Box 2.4 Steps to encourage babies to sleep through the night (Nikolopoulou and St. James-Roberts 2003)

1. Offer a regular 'focal feed' between 10.00p.m. and midnight.

2. Settle the baby into the cot to sleep and do not rock, hold or feed him just before sleeping.

3. Maximise day/night differences in the environment so as to help the baby to associate darkness with sleep by placing him to sleep in a darkened room.

4. 'Stretch' the intervals between night-time feeds once infants are growing satisfactorily beyond three weeks of age. This is to avoid linking night waking with being fed.

The authors report that this approach led to the babies being able to sleep from midnight to 5.00a.m. on at least two of three nights by eight weeks of age. They also report, however, that many parents found achieving this pattern of sleeping by their babies stressful in itself!

Other studies have explored the value of the bedtime routine. Mindell *et al.* (2009) worked with over 400 mothers and their infant or toddler children who took part in a three-week study. This showed the usefulness of a regular bedtime routine: mothers in the intervention group calmly settled their children into bed, talked or sang to them and then put out the light after 30 minutes, while mothers in the comparison group followed their usual varied practice. The routine not only resulted in significant reductions of sleeping problems for both infants and toddlers compared with those in the comparison group, but the intervention mothers also reported that their mood had improved.

SUPPORTING RECOVERY FROM PND

PND, while deeply distressing for the parent, can have a very worrying effect on young children. Babies come into the world predisposed to respond to the smiles and loving attention of their caregivers and if this is unavailable their whole development can be prejudiced. A Dutch study by Joosen *et al.* (2012) illustrates the interactive nature of smiling very clearly. This team worked with 73 mothers and their second-born children aged between three and six months. Mothers, with their infants on their laps, were asked to smile and interact joyfully face to face with their young infants for a few minutes, but then they were asked suddenly to adopt an expressionless and 'still' face for a few more minutes. Babies not only stopped smiling but were visibly distressed and confused during the period of the 'still' face (Tronick and Cohn 1989). Mothers were then encouraged to smile happily with their babies again, and in due course the babies returned their smiles[3].

The impact of the mother's 'still face' appears to be very distressing to the infant. If this 'stillness' or blank expression is all that a baby encounters with his main carer in his or her early years of life we can see how it might prejudice his or her emotional development and relationships with others. A negative, downward spiral might develop,

---

3   See *Still Face Experiment*, www.youtube.com/watch?v=apzXGEbZht0.

since the depression may in turn inhibit the processes of the mother's bonding with her baby which are so fundamental to the sense of becoming a mother. The bonding process is facilitated by the patterns of 'talk, touch and gaze' which is characteristic of parents and others interacting with small babies: talk, with expressions of admiration and amazement; touch, by the stroking and caressing of mums, dads and other relatives; and gaze by wonder-struck friends and neighbours as they encounter the new arrival.

It is possible to help mothers to notice their baby's responsiveness via Video Interactive Guidance (VIG). Using the resources of video cameras and playback machines, mothers and fathers are helped to notice the baby's giving perhaps only a fleeting smile in return for her smile. If we do not have the technical resources the same principle can be conveyed, under supervision, without a camera. We may be able to help the mother to smile at her child, even though smiling is the last thing she feels like doing. The point here is that if the mother can 'prime the pump' by regularly smiling at her child, he is highly likely to smile and return her pleasure – *even if it is feigned*. It does not seem to matter to the baby whether this smile is sincere or not – so powerful is the predisposition to return smiles to those who smile at us. We may be able to make good use of this predisposition to help a sad mother. Such an interaction can delight the mother and set in train a benign cycle of genuine smiling. The interaction will of course need to be maintained or coached for days, weeks and months, but this is one crucial way in which bonding and attachments can be strengthened.

Scott (2006 p.485) describes the process as follows:

Several studies have confirmed that the core process of sensitive responding by the parent is reliably linked to secure attachment in the child. Insensitive parenting leads to insecure attachment patterns and antisocial behaviour (Deklyen and Speltz 2001). There are several interventions that improve sensitive responding – the most effective seem to be those that include video feedback, whereby the mother watches footage of herself with her infant. The impact her overtures and responses have on her infant is drawn to her attention and feelings that get in the way are explored. The meta-analysis from the Leiden group (Bakermans-Kranenburg *et al.* 2003) reviewed over 60 randomised trials, and showed that several interventions increase sensitive responding, and that this is indeed followed by increased attachment security in the young child.[4]

If a mother, or a father, is suffering from PND, what is the research evidence about recovery? It appears that between 10 and 15 per cent of new mothers experience the disabling symptoms of PND: persisting sadness, low interest or pleasure in anything, not even the baby, together with fatigue or a sense of exhaustion. These feelings may be accompanied by broken sleep, difficulties in concentrating, poor appetite, self-blame and even thoughts of suicide. There are a number of valid and reliable scales for the measurement of PND, such as the Edinburgh Postnatal Depression Scale (EPDS) (Cox, Holden and Sagovsky 1987), but it is increasingly recommended by the National Institute for Health and Care Excellence (NICE) that mothers should be gently asked the so-called 'Whooley questions', as listed in Box 2.5.

Box 2.5 Case-finding instruments for depression (Whooley _et al._ 1997)

- During the past month, have you often been bothered by feeling down, depressed or hopeless?
- During the past month, have you often been bothered by having little interest or pleasure in doing things?
- If the woman answers 'Yes' to either of the initial screening questions a third question should be considered: 'Is this something you feel you need or want help with?'

Mann, Adamson and Gilbody (2012) suggest that if a mother responds affirmatively to one or more of these questions, it is then appropriate to ask them to complete the fuller EPDS, an instrument with ten questions which has been shown to be a valid and reliable means of identifying mothers experiencing PND.

Concerning the treatment of mild PND, one of the most encouraging bodies of evidence in this field has been provided by Holden, Sagovsky

---

4   An introduction to VIG can be seen at www.youtube.com/watch?v=DOkQladRdU.

and Cox (1989). Health visitors who had been given a manual describing PND and non-directive counselling and who had attended three weekly training sessions of two hours were able to work with 50 women who met the criteria for PND. The women were divided into a treatment group and a control group and a standardised psychiatric interview (Goldberg *et al.* 1970) and the EPND Scale were completed by all participants. The health visitors visited the women in the treatment group for an average of 8.8 visits within a mean time interval of 13 weeks and aimed to provide a confiding relationship focusing deliberately on the needs of the mother – as distinct from those of the baby, which were addressed separately. The authors reported: 'The course included instruction in counselling methods such as non-verbal encouragement and reflecting back the content of what has been said, but it was emphasised that a confiding relationship was more important than specific techniques' (Holden *et al.* 1989). At post-intervention, the scales were administered again and it was found that 18 (69%) of the mothers who had received non-directive counselling had recovered by comparison with 9 (37%) of those in the control group.

Other studies have compared the impact on PND of either antidepressant medication or community-based psychosocial support. For example, in the so-called RESPOND trial, Sharp *et al.* (2010) worked with 254 women meeting ten criteria for major depression across Bristol, south London and Manchester, who were randomly allocated to two conditions: either an antidepressant or non-directive counselling ('listening') visits. The EPDS was completed by the participants both before and after the 18 weeks of the trial. At four weeks, antidepressants were significantly more effective than supportive listening, but since by 18 weeks many of the women were receiving both forms of treatment it was difficult to distinguish between the two treatments. The authors concluded that early treatment with antidepressants leads to clinical benefit for women with PND.

So common is PND that a wide range of treatment strategies is being explored. Alongside medication and non-directive counselling, there is much interest in the potential of CBT to help women depressed following the birth of their babies. There is substantial evidence that CBT is a helpful treatment and reports of its effectiveness are widely available: for example, Milgrom *et al.* (2015). A further group of studies reported in a review by Scope *et al.* (2013) examined whether there is evidence that CBT administered in groups can be helpful for PND. The authors conclude that although the evidence available is limited, it does appear that with skilled and qualified practitioners and women's preferences for treatment being taken into account, CBT in group settings can be effective.

The overall picture appears to be that with relatively brief but specialised training, health visitors or community psychiatric nurses can help in the alleviation of PND; but that the overall management of mothers with this condition is best located with the GP, who can decide the best course of treatment in the light of local available resources, such as specially trained practitioners, and the depth of the mothers' depression.

USING IDEAS FROM CBT

One needs specialist training to practise CBT in a formal way, and we are not suggesting that volunteers or family support workers should embark on working with parents who seem to be seriously anxious or depressed. However, we are all aware of occasions when we can see that we are not thinking clearly, or that our behaviour is driving us into feeling more and more depressed. In these circumstances, in everyday life, we perhaps ring a cheerful friend or even try to detect the particular thought which triggered our sad mood, so that we can dismiss it in the light of reality. When I am feeling low, I confess I often read through appreciative reviews or evaluations of my work, which lifts my spirits. I even have a coded list of families where I know my contacts with them have made a difference to their lives or the lives of the children! 'Yes,' I say to myself, 'I know that I helped that family or that person to get over that difficulty.' If I get really low, mooning about the house reminding myself of difficulties or critical comments, I put on a Scottish dance record and the liveliness of the music and the happy associations which I bring to the Gay Gordons or Strip the Willow soon cheer me, at least temporarily.

Researchers in the field of CBT have identified a number of concepts which may lie at the heart of our sad or anxious mood, and recognising that we are rehearsing these concepts in our minds can help us stand back from them and perhaps question their accuracy.

Identifying core beliefs

A key concept which has emerged from extensive research in CBT is that we all have a number of core beliefs which are profoundly important to us. Willson and Branch (2006, p.193) describe such beliefs as follows:

> Your core beliefs are enduring ideas or philosophies that you hold very strongly and very deeply. These ideas are usually developed in childhood or early in adult life. Core beliefs are not always negative. Experiences of life and of other people generally lead to the development of healthy ideas about yourself, other people and the world... Your core beliefs are called 'core' because they're your deeply held ideas and they're at the very centre of your belief system. Core beliefs give rise to rules, demands, or assumptions, which in turn produce *automatic thoughts* (thoughts which just pop into your head when you are confronted with a situation).

If these automatic thoughts are positive and constructive, they will probably be beneficial, but if they are negative they may have destructive and sometimes lifelong effects, undermining confidence and inhibiting trust. We can all identify some of our core beliefs: some are explicitly said to us by parents or teachers, others we work out for ourselves. Statements like, 'I'm no good...my dad kept telling me so' are all too readily rehearsed; others are dismissive remarks made by parents or teachers, such as, 'You were my mistake; you shouldn't have happened' or 'You're never going to amount to anything' can blight a child's life.

Willson and Branch (2006) suggest that these core beliefs are extremely powerful; they are sometimes conscious and sometimes unconscious. Ideas which flow from them may influence all our attitudes and actions. Once aware of these beliefs, it is then sometimes possible to inspect them for accuracy or usefulness. For example, if a young woman believes that growing up in care means that she will never be able to care for a child, she may have associated ideas that she must give up her child. As a new mother, she may have come to believe that she *ought* to give up her child (Table 2.3).

Table 2.3 Example of a core belief, linked belief and negative automatic thought		
Core belief	Linked belief	Negative automatic thought
Girls who grow up in care can't look after children.	I ought to let my child be adopted.	I don't deserve this baby. I must give her up.
	I am selfish if I don't give up the baby for adoption.	She wouldn't love me. I must give her up.

This example is given to illustrate the way in which core beliefs can influence patterns of thinking almost without our being aware of the beliefs. While I am not suggesting that without appropriate training workers should involve themselves deeply in the thinking patterns of those they are trying to support, this example may prompt them to pursue training in cognitive behavioural approaches.

SUPPORTING PARENT-TO-INFANT BONDING

Increasing research attention is being devoted to the concept of bonding with the infant, whether maternal or paternal bonding. After exhaustive analysis, Bicking-Kinsey and Hupcey (2013) suggest that:

> maternal bonding may be defined as a maternal-driven process that occurs primarily throughout the first year of a baby's life, but may continue throughout a child's life. It is an affective state of the mother: maternal feelings and emotions toward the infant are the primary indicator of maternal–infant bonding…

As we saw earlier, mothers may report strong feelings of bonding and closeness toward their developing infants while in the womb, and these feelings can be reinforced by those who care for the mothers. In general, however, mothers report that they feel emotionally bonded with their newborn child at widely differing intervals after the birth: some report an instantaneous rush of love and delight upon the arrival of their infants, others say that they have never loved the child born to them, while a great many others fall between the two extremes, reporting that they *gradually* fall in love with their baby. As described above, this bonding is often conveyed through 'talk, touch and gaze', as parents interact with their babies: talking with them, cooing, whispering and murmuring to them; touching them, stroking, caressing and soothing them; and admiring, gazing and wondering at them.

The development of close emotional bonds between mothers, fathers and infants is clearly highly protective of babies' survival and appears to have evolved as parents focus intimately on his or her wellbeing. Indeed, as described, Feldman and her team (2007) have demonstrated that there is an association between the measurable level of oxytocin in the mother during pregnancy and the closeness of her bonding with the baby, as indicated by the levels of talk, touch and gaze described above. It seems that Nature intends that mothers shall 'fall in love' with their babies and that if this does not seem to be happening within a few days or weeks, then space, support and encouragement needs to be made available so that this natural relationship can be enabled to flower.

As Kennell and McGrath (2005) put it:

> Hospital staff can promote the creation of this bond by providing continuous support during labor, by placing the newborn skin-to-skin on the mother's chest immediately after delivery until the infant latches on for the first feeding, by encouraging continued breast feeding and by keeping her mother and infant always together in the first hours and days after delivery.

Herbert, Sluckin and Sluckin (1982), however, questioned the claim by Kennell and others that bonding occurs in this immediate and once-and-for-all way, and suggest that for many parents, fathers as well as mothers, it develops gradually over time. They suggest that to insist that the process is confined primarily to a period immediately after birth is to cause undue anxiety among parents who do not experience this rush of love. The evidence is, they claim, that parents need time to recover from the experience of labour, to adjust to the huge changes in their circumstances and, with support, to take responsibility for the newborn; bonding and love are then likely gradually to develop as sensitive, loving and rewarding interactions take place.

However, such bonding processes may need encouragement through the support and skilled guidance of an understanding helper. While PND and other disabling emotions can undermine the naturally developing relationship between mother, father and baby, in view of what we now understand about the plasticity of the brain, it is often possible, with skilled support, for parents actively to come to love their babies even after a clear initial rejection.

The organisation Oxpip, the Oxford Parent to Infant Project, has demonstrated that where mothers report depression and, for example, their belief that 'My baby never smiles at me', therapists using sequences of photographs can demonstrate the baby's fleeting smiles to the mother which she herself may not have noticed. From this beginning the therapists encourage interactions by the mother with her child until, typically, after some eight sessions, there is evidence of ongoing smiling between mothers and their babies. While there does not to date appear to be any randomised controlled trials confirming this process, there is abundant anecdotal evidence to support it. This exchange of affectionate expressions is the foundation of attachment, typically emanating from the baby to the mother and other caregivers. There are obviously close links between this work and that of the VIG approach, explored earlier in this chapter.

If such difficulties continue and become apparent to those trying to support them, be they lay or professional, it is usually not too late to remedy the situation. While professional help and, specifically, supervision is necessary in situations where it seems that the mother is having difficulty in bonding with her child, then Appendix 2 may be of use. This is a simple scale for mothers, or fathers, to indicate their felt level of bonding with the infant and derives from the work of Silverstein (1996). A more detailed instrument is included as Appendix 3: this is the Postpartum Bonding Instrument (Brockington 2001) and would be useful as the basis for a discussion, at the least. However, it would need a professionally qualified health practitioner to use it as a screening instrument.

ENCOURAGING FATHER INVOLVEMENT

Research into paternal–infant bonding is much more limited than that into maternal–infant relationships; however, we are seeing increasing interest in the role of fathers at all ages of the child's life. There appears, though, to be a need for far more research into father–infant bonding and father–child relationships in general. An important contribution to this field is the cross-cultural work of Veneziano (2003), which is summarised by Berk (2006, p.429) as follows:

> In studies of many societies and ethnic groups around the world, researchers coded paternal expressions of love and nurturance – evident in such behaviors as cuddling, hugging, comforting, playing, verbally expressing love, and praising the child's behaviour. Fathers' sustained affectionate involvement predicted later cognitive, emotional and social competence as strongly, and occasionally more strongly, than did mothers' warmth.

Rohner and Veneziano's study (2001) found a consistent relationship between the amount of time fathers spent near their babies and toddlers and their nurturing expressions and affection, while studies of a range of cultures found that paternal warmth protected children against an array of difficulties including emotional and behavioural problems in childhood and substance abuse and delinquency in adolescence (Grant *et al.* 2000).

A rigorous review of international studies of the impact of fathers' engagement with their young children by Sarkadi *et al.* (2008) concluded that 'active and regular engagement with the child predicts a range of positive outcomes' – where father 'engagement' is defined as direct contact such as play, reading, outings or caregiving activities. Positive long-term outcomes identified are listed in Box 2.6.

Box 2.6 Beneficial long-term outcomes of fathers' frequent involvement in the day-to-day care of their young children (Sarkadi *et al.* 2008)

- It reduces the frequency of behavioural problems in boys.
- It reduces the extent of emotional problems in young women.
- It enhances cognitive development.
- It decreases delinquency and economic disadvantage in low-income families.

More recently, Ramchandani *et al.* (2013) found evidence that engagement by fathers with their infants as young as three months may protect them from developing externalising behaviours when the toddlers are one year old. The researchers assessed the behaviour of the babies at home when they were three months old and then again at one year. They found that babies whose fathers were more involved with them in the early months, talking to them, playing with them and interacting enjoyably with them, were more manageable and had fewer behavioural upsets than did the babies whose fathers were more distant, more preoccupied with their own affairs and less interested in the child. The researchers commented: 'This association tended to be stronger for boys than for girls, suggesting that perhaps boys are more susceptible to the influence of their father from a very early age'.

The evidence, then, all points in the same direction: the involvement of fathers in bringing up their children is extremely valuable, and this involvement does not have to be at a sophisticated level. Rather, it is the engagement of fathers in the day-to-day activities of the young family, in caring for them while babies and toddlers and coping with the practicalities of bathing, feeding and changing, which appears to lay down valuable bonds of confidence and trust in the child.

ENCOURAGING BABY MASSAGE

Although the impact of baby massage has not been the focus of long-term research, there are several studies showing its benefits in the short term, particularly with preterm infants. In a rigorous review drawing on evidence from the Cochrane Database of the effectiveness of infant massage in promoting infant mental and physical health in babies under six months, Underdown *et al.* (2006) concluded that the massage had no effect on growth; however, there was 'some evidence suggestive of improved mother–infant interaction, sleep and relaxation, reduced crying and a beneficial impact on a number of hormones controlling stress… There was no evidence of effects on cognitive and behavioural outcomes, infant attachment or temperament.' These positive effects, 'improved mother–infant interaction, sleep and relaxation, and reduced crying', sound quite enough to this author to suggest that stressed parents should waste no time in learning the skills of infant massage!

Many parents begin this practice from about six weeks, when the beginnings of a routine are beginning to emerge in many families.

It is, of course, mainly mothers who practise infant massage, but there are the beginnings of an evidence base concerning fathers undertaking this role. For example, Cheng, Volk and Marini (2011) undertook a pilot study with fathers and their infants, with 12 father-and-baby pairs in the intervention group and a further 12 pairs in the comparison group. The focus was on the wellbeing of fathers rather than the babies in this study. The researchers found that 'infant massage instruction significantly decreased paternal stress', and fathers also reported enjoying opportunities to meet other fathers. While there are several examples of baby massage displayed on YouTube, Box 2.7 conveys the essentials of the process.

Box 2.7 A positive touch routine

- With the baby on his/her back, hold and stroke each hand in turn. Smile and talk softly with your baby.
- Similarly, hold and stroke each foot in turn.
- Gently stroke the face and head, especially the forehead.
- Lie the baby on his/her back on your lap with his/her head towards your knees; with the feet and legs against your tummy, stroke up the chest and across the shoulder.
- Then stroke his/her tummy in a clockwise direction.
- Lie the baby prone across your lap and stroke down his/her back and down the backs of the legs to the feet.
- Hold the baby upright against your chest and shoulder for another back rub.
- Hold the baby supported along your forearm and against your chest and gently rock.

There is an abundance of evidence demonstrating the valuable impact of infant massage on preterm babies and those with special needs as well as on the parents (see, for example, Field, Diego and Hernando-Reif 2010).

SUPPORTING THE BEGINNINGS OF INFANT-TO-PARENT ATTACHMENT

Attachment can be defined as the 'strong, affectionate tie we have with special people in our lives that leads us to feel pleasure when we interact with them and to be comforted by their nearness during times of stress' (Berk 2006). It appears that babies come into the world genetically prepared to develop this emotional tie, which emerges, typically, in the second half of the first year. There are usually understood to be four stages in its development (Box 2.8).

Box 2.8 Stages in the development of attachment (after Berk 2006)

1 Preattachment phase (birth to 6 weeks)
Infants develop the capacity to interact with those who care for them in ways which delight the caregivers: for example, at around four weeks, to return the smiles of parents and other admirers. Babies begin to recognise the smell and voice of the main caregiver, often the mother.

2 Attachment-in-the-making phase (6 weeks to 6–8 months)
Babies begin to react more confidently in the company of those who care for them most of the time and rather less confidently with less familiar carers and visitors. As they grow, learn to crawl and start to explore the world, they begin to use the mother as a secure base, widening their circle of exploration around her, but retreating to her if the world becomes suddenly alarming.

3 Main attachment phase: (6–8 months to 18–24 months).
Separation from the mother or caregiver is accompanied by protest by the toddler, indicating that the baby's security is closely linked with that person. Babies have differing temperaments, however, and not all protest to the same extent – particularly if they are accustomed to other caregivers than just the mother. Fahlberg (1988) has drawn attention to the 'hierarchy of attachment' which typically develops: that is, the baby develops bonds of security with several familiar figures in his or her circle, fathers, older brothers and sisters, grandparents and childminders, with however the preferred attachment figure, often the mother, at the top.

---

4 Development of a reciprocal relationship (18 months to 24 months and beyond)

During this time, if all goes well, the toddler's growing cognitive abilities, including language, help him or her to tolerate periods of separation. Bowlby (1979) suggested that these experiences of finding caregivers reliable and trustworthy contribute to an 'inner working model' of dependable relationships, which colour subsequent childhood and adult relationships for good or ill. Such experiences are not 'all or nothing', however: a negative experience in early life, so long as this is not too protracted, can be healed at least in part by loving and dependable relationships in later childhood or adolescence.

Much effort has been devoted to attempting to recognise and understand the patterns of attachment displayed by infants to their mothers or other main caregivers. To explore this, Ainsworth *et al.* (1978) developed the Strange Situation scenario, a setting in which babies, typically aged about one year, experience a sequence of brief separations from the mother each lasting about three minutes, as in Box 2.9.[5]

Box 2.9 Episodes in the Strange Situation scenario (Ainsworth *et al.* 1978)

1. Worker brings parent and baby to the toys in the playroom; then leaves.

2. Baby explores the toys.

3. A stranger comes in and briefly talks to the parent.

4. The parent leaves the room. If the baby is upset she tries to comfort him/her.

5. The parent returns and if the baby is upset, he/she is comforted.

6. The parent again leaves the room.

7. The stranger comes into the room again and offers comfort.

8. The parent returns and, if the baby is upset, gives comfort and introduces toys.

---

5   see *The Strange Situation*, www.youtube.com/watch?v=QTsewNrHUHU.

According to the responses of the baby to these brief periods of separation, four main groups of attachment behaviours have been noted (Box 2.10, adapted from Sharma and Cockerill 2014). For clarity, the baby is referred to as 'he' and the caregiver as 'the mother' or 'she'.

Box 2.10 Patterns of attachment (after Sharma and Cockerill 2014)

1 Secure attachment

Securely attached infants show an intimate, generally contented relationship with the parent or caregiver. They may be upset when she leaves, are happy to see her return and recover quickly from any distress. Secure infants have typically experienced sensitive and consistent parenting and so are able to use their mother as a base from which to explore. About 65 per cent of children show this pattern.

2 Insecure/avoidant attachment

About 20 per cent of infants or young children seem indifferent toward their caregiver and may even avoid her. If they get upset when alone they are comforted as easily by a stranger as by a parent.

3 Insecure/resistant attachment

About 10 per cent of infants or young children are clingy, stay close to the caregiver, get very upset when she leaves and are not comforted by strangers. They are not easily comforted and both seek comfort and resist efforts by the caregivers to comfort them.

4 Disorganised/disoriented attachment

About 15 per cent of infants or young children have no consistent way of coping with the situation of being left alone with a stranger. Their behaviour is often confused or even contradictory and they often appear disoriented, such as approaching the caregiver, but being fearful (Main and Soloman 1986).

It is this fourth group of children, those with a 'disorganised' attachment relationship, about whom there has been the greatest concern. Studies, for example by Lyons-Ruth, Bronfman and Parsons (1996), found that the mothers of children who displayed these types of attachment often had serious psychological problems and were unable to offer their children the calm and secure styles of care which contribute to security of attachment. Longitudinal studies, again by Lyons-Ruth and her collaborators, found that it was this group of children who displayed the most worrying behaviour, notably aggressiveness (Lyons-Ruth *et al.* 1999).

However, Sharma and Cockerill (2014) caution: 'A simplistic interpretation of children's attachment behaviours can do more harm than good through misattribution of causal links or consequences... Strong or weak attachment behaviours do not necessarily represent strong or weak attachments.'

Enhancing family attachment

Silverstein (1996) has made a particular study of ways of enhancing family attachment, that is, with all family members not just the main caregiver; these are relevant for all families, and would be useful for families who are fostering or adopting children. She notes that the activities involve offering reassurance, comfort, reduction of stress and shared enjoyment. They demonstrate the protection which parents can offer the child and thus clarify and strengthen the roles of all family members, the protectors and the protected. The activities are often based on some form of play which can be adapted to children of different ages and which allow them to play at the levels of younger children. For these helpful suggestions by Silverstein, see Appendix 4.

ENCOURAGING PLAY AND EARLY COMMUNICATION

A large body of research suggests that language delays can be risk factors for the development of behaviour difficulties, so it is never too early to help a toddler enjoy sounds, singing and language. Children in the first year of life are often acutely receptive to language and around the time of their first birthday they may be venturing into expressive language via babbling and echoing sounds which are part of their everyday environment.

Apart from the intrinsic satisfaction which parents can gain by beginning to interact with their baby from the very early days, this can be extremely beneficial for the infants themselves. Bidmead and

Andrews (2004) in a series of three delightful articles on enhancing parent–infant interaction have built on the understandings developed by Brazelton and Nugent (1995). They encourage their readers to show parents how early interaction with their babies is intrinsically enjoyable to both and also carries considerable additional benefits, as shown in Box 2.11.

Box 2.11 Benefits of early play (Bidmead and Mackinder 2004)

- Enhances the parent/baby relationship
- Stimulates brain development
- Raises infant self-esteem
- Raises parents' feelings of self-efficacy
- Enhances speech and language development, prerequisites for reading and writing
- Develops babies' social skills and pleasure in relationships
- Encourages development of hand–eye co-ordination.

'Play' in these early weeks and months is likely to consist mainly of smiling and nodding, soothing and singing, but as Bidmead and Mackinder note: 'When parents talk to their baby they instinctively raise and vary the tone of their voice and articulate the sound more clearly and slowly, making it far more interesting for the baby'. And they add: 'Encouraging parents to turn the television off during these times of intimate conversation means that there are less distractions for both parent and baby'.

Resources for play, speech and language development

As the baby develops, he or she will become more interested in textures, shapes and sizes and it is here that the 'treasure basket' can be a lovely resource. This can be any smooth basket or box, and can hold soft materials, natural objects such as fir cones, apples and shells without sharp edges, as well as well-washed items such as a bunch of keys or colourful plastic containers and shakers. The basket can be added to or replenished with simple, interesting items, at no cost, and if it (and other toys) is put away and brought out again after a few days, then it will have all the appeal of novelty. To have a 'special time' for mother or father to play with and sing to the baby, and to encourage brothers and sisters to take part in this special time, will all enrich these months for all concerned.

To see how babies come into the world prepared to imitate and communicate, watch *Neonate Imitation*[6] and you will see how a father seeks his baby's attention and puts out his tongue – only to have the baby, only a few hours old, imitate him and put out his own tongue! These early interactions prepare the way for fully fledged exchanges of sound and language. Moreover, infants imitate and articulate the most common sounds with astonishing accuracy.

Appendix 5 provides extremely helpful suggestions provided by the American Speech, Language and Hearing Association for encouraging speech and language at three developmental stages: from birth to two years, from two to four, and from four to six years. Helpers can make use of these suggestions for games with the children throughout the length of their contact with the children, ideally from birth throughout early childhood.

Early communication: encouraging gesturing

There is growing interest in the field of baby signing, that is, deliberately teaching certain specific gestures to babies before they can use words. Such gestures might be as shown in Box 2.12.

Box 2.12 Possible gestures, paired with words, for toddlers to convey meaning

Finger pointing to open mouth	Hungry
Patting tummy	Had enough
Hands together held to cheek	Want to sleep
Pointing to the door	Want to go out
Hands held out, palms upward	Where is…?
Hands together, then opened	Want to see book

There has been concern that teaching baby signing might impede actively learning to talk, but the evidence is to the contrary. In a major study, Goodwyn, Acredolo and Brown (2000) worked with 103 toddlers aged 11 months whom they divided into three groups: one intervention group who were taught baby signing and two control groups who were not. A range of tests were administered at 11, 15, 19, 24, 30 and 36 months to all the children. The results showed a clear advantage in terms of language development and vocabulary for the babies who had been taught signing. Other studies have achieved the same results. Deaf children already derive many benefits from learning to sign early in life: it now seems that all children can so benefit.

SUPPORT FOR PARENTS OR INFANTS WITH LEARNING DISABILITIES

These early activities will be all the more valuable if the babies show features of developmental delay or, indeed, if the parents themselves have learning disabilities and are encouraged to make an early start in stimulating their children. The positive list of items in Box 2.13 was drawn up by a gathering of parents with learning disabilities in Leeds in 2005. The earlier the support and interaction can occur, the better; the benefits will become evident in the longer term.

Box 2.13 Forms of support needed by parents with learning disabilities

- Accessible information about the parents' and baby's health and about how to look after a baby
- Self-advocacy groups (coming together with other parents)
- Getting support before things go wrong and become a crisis
- Being assessed in their own home, not in an unfamiliar residential family centre
- Assessment and support by people who understand about learning difficulties
- Advocacy

- Making courts more accessible
- Support for fathers
- Support for women and men experiencing violent relationships.

All the suggestions made above can be adapted to the circumstances of older children. It is to children in their second year of life that we now turn.

CHAPTER 3

One to Two Years

OVERVIEW

- Acknowledging risk factors
- Building on protective factors
- Supporting processes of bonding and attachment
- Accessing networks of support
- Encouraging authoritative parenting
- Using principles of social learning theory
- Encouraging cognitive and linguistic development
- Enjoying play, singing, music and movement
- Helping toddlers to develop self-control

There is of course no clear break between the first and second year of life as the baby becomes a toddler: the chapter division has been made in order to make a large amount of data manageable. The child's development continues through the chronological milestones in all respects: physiologically, emotionally, cognitively and behaviourally. In line with the previous chapter we shall briefly consider the main risks which the toddler incurs during this period, and then give far more attention to the influences and experiences which can not only offer protection against risks and hazards but also enhance development.

ACKNOWLEDGING RISK FACTORS

As established in previous chapters, environmental factors have very substantial impacts on children's behaviour. For example, a British study of over three thousand same-sex twins, both 'identical' and 'fraternal', compared the effects of the neighbourhood across six types of locality, from very disadvantaged to affluent. Results showed that children in deprived neighbourhoods were at considerably increased risk of emotional and behavioural problems, *over and above any genetic liability*. This increased risk was measurable in children as young as two years (Caspi *et al.* 2000). Other risk factors have also been identified and will be explored briefly here.

Abuse or rejection by the parent or main caregiver is of course a profoundly damaging experience for any child. He or she is totally dependent on the care of adults for very survival, and abuse of any kind, emotional, physical or sexual, together with neglect, are grounds for emergency intervention by the authorities. In the years 2013–14, in England, there were 657,800 referrals to children's social care – representing an increase of 10.8 per cent compared with the previous year. Of these, there were 142,500 enquiries within section 47 of the Children Act, an increase of 12.1 per cent over the previous year. In 2013–14, 48,300 children were the subject of a Child Protection Plan at 31 March, 2014, an increase of 12.1 per cent on 43,100 at March, 2013. Neglect and emotional abuse are the two categories that have seen the greatest increase (Department for Education 2014a).

Harsh parenting is a well-recognised ground for major concern and a recognised risk for future difficulties. We see in Table 3.1 that Baumrind (1971) has been able to distinguish several main patterns of parenting, with two key dimensions: high/low affection and warmth and high/low levels of control. Her work was developed by Maccoby and Martin (1983). High and low levels of each of these dimensions yields four main styles: authoritative, permissive, authoritarian and neglecting. The style which gives greatest cause for concern is the authoritarian, since this can readily merge into a harsh and aggressive style where the parents control their children but do so in such a way that they either fear and avoid them or react with aggression themselves. These interactions can set up ongoing conflict situations which can totally undermine the desirable loving and supportive relationships which children need from their parents. Unfortunately, these learned, harsh styles of raising children are all too often taken into the parenting practices of the next generation.

Table 3.1 The two main dimensions and four main styles of parenting (after Maccoby and Martin 1983)

	High level of warmth and acceptance	Low level of warmth and acceptance
High level of control	**Authoritative** parents tend to be high in both warmth and control, setting clear limits, expecting and reinforcing socially mature behaviour (e.g. caring for other children), but also sensitive to the child's needs. These parents are less likely to use physical punishment than more authoritarian parents. They may discipline older children by, for example, 'Time Out'. The children tend to be self-confident with high self-esteem.	**Authoritarian** parents tend to be very demanding of their children, but not to be very nurturing. They try to control their children, but give little warmth or positive attention. The children tend to react either by being fearful or by being aggressive and out of control.
Low level of control	**Indulgent, permissive** parents may not exercise necessary controls over their children. If parents are permissive towards aggression, it is likely that the children will develop aggressive behaviours.	**Neglecting, uninvolved** parents tend to be psychologically 'unavailable' to their children for a range of reasons, for example PND or being overwhelmed by other problems. The children seem to have many difficulties in relationships with adults and other children.

BUILDING ON PROTECTIVE FACTORS

Happily, in this period of one to two years both child, parents, grandparents and other people whom the toddler encounters are predisposed to make loving and intimate relationships with each other. The toddler is still wholly dependent, but not only are bonding processes usually well established in the caregivers but the whole process of attachment is deepening and becoming more precious to the child. These sequences are rooted in physiology and psychology and are clearly 'intended' by Nature as means to survival. When they go smoothly, they are wholly delightful for all concerned, but as we saw in Table 3.1 different parenting styles can markedly affect outcomes.

The role of the helping person, or family visitor, may well be to foster both bonding in the caregivers and attachment in the toddler.

SUPPORTING PROCESSES OF BONDING AND ATTACHMENT
Supporting bonding

We encountered the terms 'bonding' and 'attachment' in Chapter 2. Here we wish to confirm that whereas formerly the term 'attachment' was sometimes used loosely and interchangeably for all relationships between infants and their parents, increasingly, 'bonding' is used to refer to the parent-or-other-caregiver-to-infant relationship, while 'attachment' refers to the emotional link between the infant and parents and caregivers.

As we saw in the previous chapter, the processes whereby babies come into the world prepared to make close and affectionate relationships with those who care for them are of the greatest importance. If things go well, this intimate and loving tie develops spontaneously, with the main carers becoming closely bonded with the child as they interact with him or her on a day-by-day basis and the child becoming securely attached to the caregivers, gaining confidence thereby to test out the world. A highly important film made in 1952 by James Robertson demonstrated the impact of admitting young children to hospital with little or no visiting allowed by parents. The film changed medical and hospital policy on this issue and brought about sweeping changes [7]However, some parents find it very hard to provide the ongoing sensitive care which their child needs in these early dependent months and years. This may be because they genuinely do not understand the desirability of a fairly consistent and dependable relationship between themselves and their babies or toddlers; it may be because they themselves had difficult experiences in their own earliest years; or it may be because they are preoccupied with their own problems such as the care of other children. I was fortunate enough to be present when a toddler who had been in the care of foster parents was gradually being reintroduced to the care of her mother during a contact visit. This mum had had

---

7   See *A Two Year Old Goes to Hospital*, www.youtube.com/watch?v=s14Q-_Bxc_U.

PND and had been unable to care for her little girl, feeling distant and detached from her, but was now rather better. The toddler, however, had naturally become very attached to the foster parents and it took weeks of carefully planned meetings between foster mother, natural mother and toddler before the little one allowed herself to be cared for by her own mother. Skilled and sensitive care continued from the foster mother, the social worker as well as the birth mother who were present at all the contact meetings; over many weeks the birth mother gradually gained the toddler's confidence, and it was a delight to see first the renewal of contact between mother and child and then the growing affection between the them as the two played together and developed close relationships. Eventually, after many months of supervised contact, the birth mother said that she had 'fallen in love again' with her little girl and, later still, the toddler went to live permanently with her at their home.

Supporting attachment

The evidence that a strained or insecure attachment in children of this age can be built or rebuilt is demonstrated by the success of a great many fostering and adoptive relationships. A major study undertaken by researchers at Bristol University (Selwyn, Wijedasa and Meakings 2014) analysed national data on 37,335 adoptions of children over 12 years and found that only 3.2 per cent of children moved out of their adoptive homes prematurely. If children did not have their main attachment needs met through fostering or adoption, far more would fail. The strategies suggested by Silverstein for fostering attachment, already referred to and which are given in Appendix 4, are invaluable and can readily be adapted for toddlers.

While attachment processes begin in the first year of life, the second year of life is the one during which they become particularly significant. The toddler's sense of security is usually closely linked with the availability of the mother or main caregiver, although if he has been cared for regularly by other family members, childminders or nursery staff, they are likely to be able to soothe him in times of difficulty or distress.

If the child is to be looked after by a childminder or attends a nursery on a full-time or part-time basis it is normally important that the parent introduces the toddler to his or her key worker gradually, for an hour or two a day over several days and weeks, until the child has learned to trust this alternative caregiver and, gradually, other nursery staff. It is counter-productive to try to rush this stage. It is desirable too that the same person should collect the toddler on each occasion, so that the child learns that a few key people provide security. It is also helpful if a simple routine can be followed on reaching home, perhaps ten or fifteen minutes on the parent's lap to calm the child and settle him or her down. Many toddlers will want their 'snuggy' or favourite soft toy to cuddle and to self-soothe – to help them relax and to comfort themselves before rejoining the hurly burly of family life.

Encouraging positive feedback: dual advantages

The seminal studies of Hart and Risley (1995) are extremely important here: these researchers monitored a cross-section of children in respect of their language and social experience from the age of eight months to two and a half years and found that 'the amount of children's experience with encouraging feedback was strongly associated with the magnitude of their accomplishments at age 3 and at age 9–10.' In other words, children who receive little encouragement or even none at all are seriously at risk of underachieving and of being unable to make the most of their potential.

Positive feedback has another advantage, however, especially with young children: it reassures them that the person caring for them cherishes them and wishes to nurture them. This in turn reassures them, makes them feel secure and strengthens the attachment to the parent or caregiver. In one of my research studies, a little girl was displaying seriously difficult behaviour: I was able to teach the mother to notice the little girl's positive behaviours and to praise her for them. The mother later reported with delight, 'She gives me a love – more affectionate. She will sit on my knee with her arms around me. My husband says she seems completely different' (Sutton 2001).

ACCESSING NETWORKS OF SUPPORT

The network of Children's Centres set up across the UK offers an amazing resource for lonely or inexperienced parents and families.

Although a substantial number of individual Centres have closed because of national and local economic difficulties, most localities still have a web of Centres available for at least several sessions a week. These are literally open to everyone, staffed by trained and sensitive workers who are committed to young children and their families. The Centres are cheerful, welcoming places, where all parents and young children can rely on friendly staff and a wide range of people to talk to; they are wonderfully equipped and a range of activities for children and parents is offered by specialised staff.

In order to encourage parents to use Children's Centres, in some places now renamed Children, Young People and Families Centres, several key services are often made available there: health visitors may locate clinics for weighing and monitoring child development; speech and language therapists hold sessions there; play workers engage toddlers and parents in simple interactive fun with sand, water, clay and craftwork which can then be practised at will at home. I cannot speak too highly of the programme of singing, creative play and story-telling together with physical activities which I observed when I was a volunteer at our local Children's Centre. With attentive staff, really concerned to make parents and children from a range of cultural and linguistic groups welcome, and magnificent play equipment such as tricycles, scooters and balls of every size and colour readily available for indoor or outdoor play according to the season, I wished that such resources had been available when my own children were small! If, for whatever reason, parents do not wish or are not in a position to make use of Children's Centres, there is typically a wide range of resources for young children in libraries, playgroups and in the homes of childminders.

ENCOURAGING AUTHORITATIVE PARENTING

The style of parenting which a child experiences contributes very substantially to his or her wellbeing. Longitudinal studies have shown that just as harsh, humiliating and punitive parenting is a major risk factor for subsequent antisocial behaviour, so firm, authoritative parenting is a protection against such hazards. These styles of parenting are shown above in Table 3.1.

So, how do we help parents practise authoritative methods of bringing up their children? It is highly desirable that all those who care for the child should be in broad agreement about the routine the child should follow, and which patterns of behaviour are or are not allowed. I recall very clearly one of the children with whose family I worked where this had not been done. The little boy, let's call him Robin, was two and a half and a big child for his age. He was dearly loved by his mother and stepfather and by the members of his extended family. Every Saturday morning he visited his Uncle Bill who lived nearby. Bill also loved Robin and wanted to give him a happy time, so he had taught Robin rough and tumble play and, as he got older, how to play-fight; the two spent nearly the whole of every Saturday morning in rough and tumble play on the rug – and they both enjoyed themselves hugely. The trouble was that Robin, now a very strong and confident little boy, took his newly acquired patterns of play to the two Stay and Play groups he attended with his mother and to the story-time session at the library. It was not long before he began to use his strength to get hold of any toy, particularly tricycles, which other children had but which he wanted – to the indignation of the parents of the children who gave way before Robin's onslaught. The complaints about Robin flooded in and it was not long before his parents were asked not to bring him to the groups any more. Consternation at home!

Now Robin's mother and stepfather were mild and peaceable people, and they had noticed that Robin was particularly hard to manage after the Saturday mornings with Uncle Bill. Robin was also becoming increasingly cheeky at home; I was asked to advise them how to proceed. Robin's Mum found her brother a bit daunting and didn't want to stop the Saturday morning visits but when my assessment showed that it was very likely that Robin was simply following what Uncle Bill had taught him, they realised there had to be changes. Fortunately, Robin's step-dad was willing to explain to Uncle Bill that either he substituted some other activities for rough and tumble, and refuse all demands from Robin to fight, or the visits would have to stop. There was a row, but the step-dad held firm and gradually as trips to the park were arranged on Saturday mornings, play-fighting was phased out and aggressiveness was handled firmly, Robin's behaviour calmed down. He was told that any times when he played calmly for fifteen minutes with other children would be rewarded with a sticker on his chart; five stickers on any one day meant he could play a card game with both Mum and Dad before bed. However, any instances of hitting or snatching toys would mean that he would be taken home immediately. Within a month, Robin was readmitted to his Stay and Play groups and had to be taken home only once. The data from this example is incorporated in my research papers (Sutton 1992, 1995).

So we can turn now to social learning theory, an illuminating body of ideas, grounded in abundant research.

USING PRINCIPLES OF SOCIAL LEARNING THEORY

It is essential that any helping person, professional or lay, should have a good understanding of this body of concepts. It is highly desirable too that parents should know of the principles because they are operating all about us, whether we appreciate it or not.

Modelling

This refers to the natural process whereby children learn by observing the behaviours and attitudes of those about them, and copying them. Family life provides a natural setting for children to observe their parents and other adults and use them, for good or ill, as models to imitate. During the second year of life, when toddlers typically spend a good deal of time with their parents and caregivers, these people, whether they realise it or not, are models of behaviour which will influence children throughout their lives. Berk (2006) suggests that certain characteristics in those caring for children make it more likely that those children will copy these models (Box 3.1).

> **Box 3.1 Characteristics of those caring for children which make it more likely that children will imitate them (Berk 2006)**
>
> - *Warmth and responsiveness.* Personal warmth seems to make children, particularly preschool children, more attentive and receptive to the model.
> - *Competence and power.* Children inevitably attend to competent and powerful people in their environments – who thus act as models for behaviour, for good or ill.
> - *Consistency between what is said and what is done.* If those who are chosen as models actively 'practise what they preach', then children experience consistent examples of how to behave with minimal conflict between word and deed. If there is conflict, the action is more likely to be imitated than the word.

If parents are concerned about their toddler's behaviour it may be possible to sit down with them and explore what is worrying them. Often these may be feelings that the child 'is naughty', or that he 'doesn't take notice of what he is told to do'. Sometimes giving information about age-appropriate behaviour for a toddler of 18 months will be sufficient to reassure them: a copy of *Mary Sheridan's From Birth to Five Years* (updated by Sharma and Cockerill 2014) is invaluable for supplying this information in very accessible ways.

Reinforcement and feedback

As I have written earlier (Sutton 2006), there is no doubt that parents, childminders, playgroup leaders, teachers and all those who take care of children wittingly or unwittingly practise the principles of reinforcement: 'You came when I called, Danny. Good boy!'; 'You brought me the nappy, Molly. Thank you so much!'; 'When you've eaten your chapatti, Usha, you can have some fruit.'

Positive reinforcement/feedback (reward)

This is any event which has the effect of increasing the probability of the behaviour which preceded it occurring again: for example, appreciation, praise, recognition, pay packets and salaries. A child commended for trying hard at her school work is likely to continue to try hard. An employee who receives a bonus in her pay packet with appreciation of how she has helped to meet the company's targets is likely to continue to work to that end. The power of positive reinforcement, sometimes loosely called positive feedback, is only gradually becoming understood by the general public – which is a great pity as it can contribute to the resolution of so many interpersonal difficulties. However, it is worth stating again the most effective procedure for giving praise to children (Box 3.2).

Box 3.2 Effective procedures for giving praise or positive feedback to children (Blaze *et al.* 2014)

Praise should be:

- contingent upon behaviour
- specific, to help the child know which behaviour is being commended
- immediate
- effort-based, relating to the child's trying to achieve something.

Negative reinforcement/feedback

This is, technically, any happening which, because it is unpleasant, such as the noise of a pneumatic drill, has a rewarding effect when it stops. In popular usage, however, negative reinforcement or feedback often means a penalty.

Penalty/punishment/sanction

This is any event which has the effect of decreasing the probability of the behaviour which preceded it happening again: for example, criticism, blame, being ignored. A child whose efforts to use a spoon or other eating equipment are criticised or ignored is unlikely to continue to try, while a child who is told she is too messy to feed herself may come to expect to be fed for months or even years. For some children, however, any attention, even being scolded or smacked, is better than none, so *an apparent punishment may in fact be a reward.*

The patterns of reinforcement and their effects are summarised in Box 3.3.

Box 3.3 Patterns of reinforcement and their effects (Herbert 1987)

Desirable behaviour + reinforcement → more desirable behaviour

Desirable behaviour + no reinforcement → less desirable behaviour

Undesirable behaviour + reinforcement → more undesirable behaviour

Undesirable behaviour + no reinforcement → less undesirable behaviour

---

The above relationships between a behaviour and what comes afterwards are happening all around us. We have only to watch patiently and we shall see them.

Behaviour analysis

It is extremely valuable throughout childhood for parents and carers to have sufficient understanding of these key theoretical ideas concerning behaviour for them to be able to understand the context of many children's difficult conduct – so as to nip it in the bud. Accordingly, I give here a way of looking at common behaviours which parents often complain about. I call it the A-B-C sequence: A stands for 'Activator' or 'Antecedent', B for 'Behaviour' and C for 'Consequence'.

The A-B-C sequence

The sequence indicates that behaviour does not ordinarily happen in isolation – or 'out of the blue'. Usually the child will have a motive for behaving as he or she does, and often it will be to gain attention.

Sometimes this attention is urgently needed for their overall wellbeing; at other times it is not, but it is enjoyable to the child to be noticed and to receive that attention. Usually, there will be an event or action which is an immediate activator or antecedent of the behaviour and another event or action which takes place as a consequence of the behaviour.

To help you gain confidence in looking at some difficulties as an A-B-C sequence, Table 3.2 shows some examples which parents have noticed. They may be familiar!

Table 3.2 The A-B-C analysis of some behaviours		
Activator/Antecedent	Behaviour	Consequence
Anna was having breakfast.	She kept getting down from her seat.	Mum followed her round with a bowl of cereal, feeding her spoonfuls.
Sunil was told to leave the TV off.	He kept putting it on.	In the end it was left on, 'to give people a bit of peace'.
Delroy wanted to go to the swings. Dad said it was too late.	Delroy lay on the floor and kicked and screamed.	Dad gave way. They went to the swings and were back late.
James wanted an ice cream while out shopping. Mum said 'No'.	James yelled and called his mother a 'horrible old cow'.	Mum gave way, because she was embarrassed at how people looked at her.

You can see that in the above examples the Consequence, what followed the child's Behaviour, was that he or she was rewarded by getting his or her own way. In other words, the child received positive reinforcement (reward) for behaving in a difficult way – which made it all the more likely to happen again.

Now let's have a look at examples of how A for Activator or Antecedent can result in certain behaviours.

Activator/Antecedent	Behaviour	Consequence
The health visitor asked Sally to draw a picture. Mum said, 'She won't; she's shy.'	Sally had reached for the crayon, but when she heard what Mum said, she drew back her hand.	The health visitor was unable to persuade her to take the crayon and draw.
Mum had been trying to help Jack to go to sleep without his dummy. Dad was putting Jack to bed. He said, 'Are you sure you can manage without your dummy?'	Jack whined and grizzled and cried for his dummy.	Dad gave Jack his dummy. It was weeks before Mum tried again to help him give it up.

In these examples, Mum's and Dad's words are acting as the Activator or trigger to the Behaviour. The children are effectively being cued, or coached, to behave in an anxious way or undesirable way – probably contrary to the actual wishes of their parents.

My colleague Di Hampton points out that if we want children or young people's behaviour to change then two actions need to take place:

- Parents or caregivers need to change their behaviour; that is, do something different.

- The activator and/or the consequence needs to change as these are the events which keep the unwanted behaviour going.

Talking about parents' feelings around changing behaviour

Several studies have shown that although many parents do not have an understanding of the idea of reinforcement and that unwittingly they are often rewarding the very behaviour they are complaining of; others do understand this but cannot bring themselves to be – as they see it – really strict with their child. Scott (2006, p.486) describes this common situation as follows:

> Certainly in clinical practice it seems helpful actively to solicit what parents are feeling as well as helping them to develop skills to change relationships. For example, not infrequently parents have difficulties setting limits and fail to follow through despite repeated practice. Sensitive exploration of their beliefs sometimes reveals that they themselves were brought up in a painfully harsh way, so they shy away

from almost any discipline at all since the last thing they want to do is to make their child suffer as they did. Helping them understand and experience through role-play that gentle but firm parenting is not abusive can then lead to progress.

In another situation, I remember one mother whose toddler didn't allow her a moment to herself, even to go to the toilet, so closely did he cling to her. She told me that as a child she had felt ignored by her parents. She determined she would never ignore her own child, so she didn't: she never asked him to wait, or did something else before attending to his requests. She was, unwittingly, rewarding him repeatedly for pestering her – so he went on doing it! Talking for a little while about her feelings as a child at being ignored and explaining how her situation had developed was sufficient to free her from guilt at ignoring her child's demands as necessary and to work out with me how to achieve some time for herself.

Other parents may have a 'precious child', that is, a long-awaited child, or one born after a bereavement during a previous pregnancy. These parents are understandably so anxious about their child that they find it almost impossible to deny him anything or even to let him become frustrated. Of course, in such circumstances, preliminary time must be spent in ensuring that they receive counselling or bereavement support so that they can deal with the intense anxiety which they feel when having to say 'No' to their toddler and withstand his protests.

Maintaining 'good' behaviour

I have dealt with this issue in some depth in my book *Helping Families with Troubled Children* (Sutton 2006) but, in brief, there are several strategies for this, all flowing naturally from social learning theory:

- The simplest is to commend the child for behaving in the desired way; that is, as suggested above, 'You came when I called Jack; well done!' or 'You've eaten up all your dinner! That is so good.'

- It helps if a little child can learn 'family rules', routines for doing things which happen almost every day, such as arrangements for meals, for getting up in the morning and going to bed at night, for going out and coming in and for making visitors to the house welcome. These are often implicit, rather than spelled out, but they happen so often that children learn them by 'osmosis'.

- If necessary, for these tiny children, a mild penalty can be administered: a firm 'No!' is usually enough to convey disapproval of unwanted behaviour, such as slopping food, throwing toys or other objects or hitting other children. But a minute, or at the most two minutes, sitting on a cushion or mat facing the wall and being ignored during that time is usually sufficient for one- and two-year-olds to understand that throwing food or hitting other children is *not* acceptable.

Cognitive processes

As well as modelling themselves on influential figures around them and responding to patterns of reinforcement by those who care for them, toddlers and small children as they develop are beginning to remember previous outcomes, to recall different responses by different caregivers and to initiate activities which meet their needs or wishes. For example, a toddler, remembering that Granny often comes to the house with a bag of sweets, may learn to greet her not with a hug but with an enquiry for 'fweeties?'; another toddler may have learned very early in life to play off one parent against another, and so rushes off with 'Me ask Daddy!' about a request which has already been refused by Mum – because the two parents have not worked out a common decision on this issue; while a third, found to be missing for a few minutes, may be discovered next door in the search for 'choccy', recently enjoyed there.

A good grasp of all these theoretical points on the part of practitioners or other helpers can be of enormous usefulness in helping parents to understand patterns of behaviour which can seem incomprehensible to them – as well as how best to react. For example, if a toddler has learned a wide range of swear words and is beginning to enjoy the effect of using these in public settings, it is really *not* a good idea to laugh at this behaviour or to tell neighbours about it in his hearing. The toddler will be echoing (modelling) words which he has heard and his undesirable behaviour is being reinforced by the amused responses of the adults who hear the story.

Helping families make use of these ideas

This second year of life is a good time to help parents set up desired patterns of behaviour for their toddlers. Berk (2006) describes how, between 12 and 18 months, toddlers begin to show the first glimmerings of self-control, and she comments that at this age: 'Toddlers start to show clear awareness of caregivers' wishes and expectations and can obey simple requests and commands... Compliance quickly leads to toddlers' first conscience-like verbalizations – for example, correcting herself by saying, "No, can't," before touching a delicate object or jumping on the sofa (Kochanska 1993).'

This, then, is a good time for parents to begin to be aware of how simple house rules can provide useful guidance for their developing toddlers. It helps a lot if these house rules can be worked out by or with both parents and shared with others who have the care of the child, such as childminders, grandparents and aunts and uncles. These people may disagree with a guideline such as 'Only one sweetie a day' or 'We stay upstairs after washing or a bath', but if parents practise the rules and ask grandparents and childminders to do the same, they can soon become established in the family routine. In this connection, I have written a short poem entitled 'A Child's Spirit', which is included as Appendix 6.

We have written elsewhere (Sutton and Herbert 2008) that this is the age when parents and caregivers might offer children '5 praises a day'– echoing the encouragement which we all receive to eat five fruit and vegetables portions a day. Such a practice is well grounded in theory and evidence (Box 3.4). Appendix 7 illustrates the card which has been distributed widely in Leicester and Leicestershire, the impact of which is currently being evaluated.

One of the main instruments which my colleague Sue Westwood and I are using to evaluate the impact of the '5 Praises a Day' study is the Strengths and Difficulties Questionnaire (SDQ) (Goodman 1987). This wonderful instrument, which is tailored to the circumstances of children aged 2–4, 4–10 and 11–17, is composed of 25 questions, divided into 5 subscales: the child's strengths, his or her emotional difficulties, hyperactivity and relationships with peers. It has formats for completion by parents as well as teachers, together with a format for completion by young people themselves in the 11–17 age range. Further, it has formats for both pre- and post-intervention and has been translated into no fewer than 80 languages. Finally, in a gesture of wonderful generosity, the authors have made this admirable instrument available for downloading from the Internet! I commend it to readers and practitioners alike with all my heart.

Box 3.4 Theoretical principles underpinning the '5 praises a day' approach

- It strengthens pleasurable attachment to parents or those who care for them.
- It clarifies for the child what behaviours are expected of him or her by parents.
- It gives the child positive reinforcement (reward) for these behaviours.
- It ensures that children receive plenty of encouragement each day.

The importance of early encouragement contrasted with the impact of being ignored or receiving little or no positive feedback has been clearly demonstrated in the research of Hart and Risley (1995). These researchers gathered information over about two and a half years from 13 professional families, 23 working class families and 6 families receiving welfare benefits. They recorded the interactions between parents and children aged 10 months to 36 months for an hour every month, noting the number of words used, the vocabulary and the types of feedback given to children. We shall consider the results concerning language development below, but at this point it is the data concerning encouragements and discouragements which call for urgent attention. Table 3.3 shows the results.

Table 3.3 Experiences of average encouragements and discouragements across three types of family within a year (Hart and Risley 1995)

	Encouragements	Discouragements
Professional family	166,000	26,000
Working-class family	62,000	36,000
Family on welfare	26,000	57,000

This study demonstrates the processes, or some of them, which contribute so much to the advantages of children from professional families. As I have written earlier (Sutton 2006): 'And of what do these underpinning processes consist? They are not all that difficult to provide for every child: they are language baths, given through conversations, stories, poems and song; they are frequent doses of nurturance, affection and encouragement and they are generous offerings of admiration and praise – all administered daily from infancy!'

Finally in this section, Box 3.5 summarises the principles of cognitive behavioural theory.

Box 3.5 Summary of principles of cognitive behavioural theory (after Martin and Pear 1992)

1. A behaviour that is rewarded is more likely to be repeated.

2. A behaviour that is penalised is less likely to be repeated.

3. A behaviour that is consistently ignored or penalised is likely to fade away.

4. A behaviour that has been established, then ignored, then rewarded again, is likely to start all over again.

5. A behaviour may be learned because it occurs in association with another behaviour.

6. A behaviour may be learned by imitating another's behaviour.

7. A behaviour may be acquired by thinking it through and practising it beforehand.

8. A belief can be examined to see if it is based on sound evidence.

9. Beliefs can be tested out to see if they are accurate or not.

10. People can be helped to use problem-solving skills rather than 'rehearsing the problem'.

ENCOURAGING COGNITIVE AND LINGUISTIC DEVELOPMENT
Enhancing young children's intelligence

There is, unfortunately, much evidence that many children and young people who find themselves in trouble with the law have not reached their cognitive potential. This means that these children are not able to take full advantage of the resources of education and may be inclined, as they get older, to truant from a school programme which they find difficult or which they see as irrelevant. One of the objectives of several initiatives focused on children's early experience has been to raise their cognitive abilities.

Accordingly, there has been extensive research into ways of enhancing children's cognitive potential; that by Protzko, Aronson and Blair (2013) is a recent example of this. These authors conducted 'meta-analyses', gathering data on as many well-designed studies as they could find in the field in question, and drew out conclusions from literally thousands of investigations. They identified four clusters of interventions which led to significantly enhanced intelligence in the children taking part in the study (Box 3.6).

Box 3.6 Strategies found to enhance young children's intelligence (Protzko, Aronson and Blair 2013)

- Supplementing young children's diets with long-chain polyunsaturated fatty acids (fish oil).
- Enrolling children in early educational interventions.
- Reading to children in an interactive manner; that is, talking about the story.
- Sending children to preschool. Here the authors noted that ' ... preschools which included a specific language-development component were found to be somewhat more effective at raising IQ'.

It will be evident from this and other reports that encouraging talking, conversation, singing and using language in fun ways at home, at nursery and in preschool is a fundamental strategy for enhancing cognitive abilities. It follows that it is very beneficial if parents, grandparents and all who care for young children talk clearly, frequently and engagingly to them. We explore this idea below.

Encouraging talking

I recall a mother who, when I asked if she talked much to her two-year-old said, 'No I don't talk to him. He hasn't learned to talk yet.' So, it is still not common knowledge that children learn to speak by being spoken to, and that they can acquire large vocabularies and greater understanding just by hearing the words used by those about them. Certain home circumstances have been identified as enhancing children's cognitive and linguistic development, as shown in Table 3.4.

Table 3.4 Features of home life which contribute to enhancing children's cognitive and linguistic development (after Bradley *et al.* 2001)

Infancy and toddlerhood	Early childhood	Middle childhood
• Emotional and verbal responsiveness of the parent • Parental acceptance of the child • Parental involvement with the child • Organisation of the physical environment • Provision of appropriate play materials • Variety in daily stimulation	• Parental pride, affection and warmth • Avoidance of physical punishment • Language stimulation • Stimulation of academic behaviour • Stimulation through toys, games and reading material • Parental modelling and encouragement of social maturity • Variety in daily stimulation • Physical environment: safe, clean and conducive to development	• Emotional and verbal responsiveness of the parent • Emotional climate of the parent–child relationship • Parental encouragement of social maturity • Provision for active stimulation • Growth-fostering materials and experiences • Family participation in developmentally stimulating experiences • Parental involvement in child-rearing • Physical environment: safe, clean and conducive to development

It is noteworthy how often the word 'stimulation' and the phrase 'language stimulation' appear. Language is an absolutely primary vehicle for children's development.

The bedtime story

I have given this topic its own section because its importance, both emotionally and in terms of language development, is so compelling. Duursma, Augustyn and Zuckerman (2008, p.556), in a detailed paper, summarise the research evidence for the value of reading to children in general:

> Reading aloud to young children, particularly in an engaging manner, promotes emergent literacy and language development and supports the relationship between parent and child. In addition it can promote a love for reading which is even more important than improving specific literacy skills.

Other researchers have demonstrated that tiny children, as young as eight months, have been found to show an interest in books when their parents look at them and talk about the pictures with them; and this interest increases as the child develops, during the second and later years of childhood. Without formal teaching, little children learn to recognise letter shapes and to see how they can be linked with other letter shapes, be this in English or a range of other languages. They acquire vocabulary painlessly and many studies show that children who are read to during the preschool years move into reading with greater ease than those who have not had this opportunity. They also do better in language development in the later years of primary school. So reading to children is an activity that any adult, parent, relative or home visitor can enjoy, knowing that it contributes substantially to the child's development as well as being a positive activity in its own right.

How I, as an eight-year-old in a small village school in Wiltshire in the 1940s, looked forward to Friday afternoons, when our hardworking schoolmaster, Mr Webb, sole teacher of a class of 30 boys and girls aged 7 to 13, used to read *The Wind in the Willows* to us! I absolutely loved this story, have read it to my grandchildren, and it has remained one of my beloved books throughout my life.

And reading of course supports relationships: if being read to in almost any context is enriching, how much more so is being read to at bedtime! The time that it takes to read a story, perhaps around 10–15 minutes, not only provides a comforting routine but also a chance for the child to calm down physically in the care of a familiar adult, often a parent. The shared enjoyment of the stories and the warmth and security of the bedtime routine in a loving relationship often stand out when adults look back on their childhood memories.

Further ways of promoting children's cognitive and linguistic development

Many examples are included in Appendix 5, drawn from the American Speech, Language and Hearing Association, but I give below some additional strategies which have been found valuable. These can be used for toddlers in the second year of life, but can also be adapted for older children:

- Treasure baskets: these contain everyday items which a toddler can play with alone, or which can be talked about with a caregiver.

- Pots and pans from the kitchen, with lids and a wooden spoon. The toddler can amuse himself for long stretches of time putting pots one into another and banging them with a wooden spoon.

- Musical sounds: a simple wooden xylophone can provide a wide range of experience and contribute to a sensitivity to sounds.

Intensive early education

There seems to be a natural aversion to 'pressurising' children to acquire knowledge and skills early in their lives: we are reluctant to push them into premature learning and we cite Scandinavian experience which shows that children who start formal education far later than in the UK are able to demonstrate the same levels of knowledge and skill as British children who normally start formal school at the age of four or five.

However, it is important to take note of the research concerning the early education of young children, such as that offered by Montessori approaches.

For example, He *et al.* (2009) compared the effects of Montessori education and traditional education on the intellectual development in children aged two to four years. Children whose intelligence growth levels were similar at the outset of the study were randomly allocated to one or other of the two modes of education. Both groups of children received the traditional education, but the Montessori group experienced two hours of specific Montessori activities daily. It was found, after one year, that the levels of performance of children in the Montessori education group were significantly higher than those in the traditional education group in the following areas: gross motor ability, fine motor ability, language, adaptability and social behaviour development.

With such evidence of the effectiveness of Montessori education in so many different areas, policy makers should surely promote extensive training of teachers and classroom assistants in, or at least in line with, this widely respected approach – and in others which can demonstrate such impressive evidence of effectiveness. While it is not intended to suggest that home visitors should or could emulate the work of trained Montessori teachers, this evidence demonstrates that children, particularly young children, are eminently responsive to experiences which enhance their language, their fine and gross motor skills and their social behaviour. In other words, their genetic inheritance can be developed and their potential enhanced by formal and informal experiences – at home or in nursery or playgroup. This seems to be particularly important for children coming from poor backgrounds, for while, as we saw above, the progress achieved by children in attending Children's Centres is to be warmly welcomed, the closure of many of these Centres is threatening a wonderful resource and all that can be offered there.

A related paper by Howe (1990) addresses the issue of the effectiveness of intensive early education. He suggests that parents are confused and bewildered by the contradictory messages from specialists in this field: on the one hand some experts tell them that intensive early education can elicit very high levels of intelligence and ability but others claim that such levels are associated only with very favourable innate endowment. Howe examines both positions and arrives at the following conclusion: '...there does exist a substantial body of empirical evidence pointing firmly to the conclusion that for most if not all children, with careful and imaginative use of the resources that are available to parents, the scope for increased and accelerated early progress is truly enormous.'

I emphasise this point not because I am trying to put an extra load on already stressed families and 'blame' them for their children's difficulties, but because there is a lot at stake and if nursery nurses or home visiting volunteers can stimulate young children in an ethical and light-hearted way, with games, conversation and fun, this can be invaluable. In view of the evidence that low intellectual attainment is a major risk factor for children having difficulties in meeting their potential in school and in the adult world, we need to take account of firm and reliable evidence to enhance children's wellbeing and that in the field of extending cognitive potential is particularly important.

In this connection it is of great interest that children of two years of age are now eligible to attend Children's Centre activities in England for fifteen hours weekly at no charge – a significant change of policy in this area.

ENJOYING PLAY, SINGING, MUSIC AND MOVEMENT

What I have written above may seem very solemn and intense. Now it is time to draw attention to the importance of play, fun, games and music in bringing up young children. Because play and fun are intrinsically enjoyable, it is not usually difficult to find activities which bring smiles of pleasure and delight to young children. Initially, very simple games and rhymes will engage them and make them laugh, such as:

Peep-bo! (Peekaboo!)

Where's it gone? Searching... No... No... No... No... There it is!

Nursery rhymes with actions: Twinkle, twinkle little star...

Round and round the garden...

Row, row, row your boat...

One, two, three, four, five... Once I caught a fish alive...

Clapping to music and to nursery rhymes.

Putting 'Laughing babies' into a search engine will lead to a delightful display of babies laughing at the most unsophisticated of activities: let's follow their example.

Many children enjoy rough and tumble play too, as when Dad chases them round the room on all fours and then rolls them over and over when he catches them. This is *not* best enjoyed just before bedtime!

Outdoor play in gardens and parks gives scope for extensive physically active play – particularly good for soaking up the energies of very lively children. A trip to the park, even on a dull and miserable day, is often worth the trouble of getting dressed in jackets and wellies, so a family helper or home visitor who takes the children out on a chilly afternoon is making a blessed contribution to family life. If she talks to them as they go along, this will be invaluable, even though no one may appreciate just how much she is contributing!

HELPING TODDLERS TO DEVELOP SELF-CONTROL

Children's ability to practise self-control is a fairly new field of psychological research, but one which is attracting increasing attention. One of the originators of this field is Walter Mischel who, working with large numbers of young children, offered them a choice: he placed marshmallows, a favourite sweet, in front of them and told them they could either have those sweets immediately or, if they waited some non-specified time, they could have twice that number of marshmallows. On following all these children up later in their childhood, Mischel, Mishoda and Rodriguez (1989) found that those who managed to 'delay gratification', that is, to wait longer for more sweets, were those children who became more conscientious, more persistent and eventually more successful in their school careers. It appears that the ability to delay gratification, which can be learned, is an extraordinarily useful characteristic! It was one of the early studies in self-control, although it was not appreciated as such at the time.

Moffitt *et al.* (2011) have been deeply involved in a New Zealand study of 1000 children from birth to age 32 years, the Dunedin Study, monitoring their development against a wide range of characteristics. One of the objectives of the study was to enhance the children's cognitive abilities, but the data showed that this was not achieved. However, there were other unexpected positive outcomes. Some of the children demonstrated lower levels than others of dropping out of school, of teenage pregnancy, of becoming offenders and of work absenteeism. When the common element characterising all these children was sought and identified it was found that they had high levels of self-control, illustrated by conscientiousness, self-discipline and perseverance. The data also showed that high levels of self-control in childhood were associated in adulthood with good physical health, relative freedom from substance abuse, competence in managing personal finances and avoidance of involvement in offending.

This team pointed out that self-control is an 'umbrella construct' with immediate associations with several disciplines; it is involved in the development not only of characteristics such as conscientiousness but also delay of gratification, willpower, and control of hyperactivity and impulsivity. Children who can control impulses and cope with being denied immediate reward are often those who go on to enjoy success in school and adult life. Research continues about the age(s) at which these characteristics should be inculcated.

So how should parents and those who support parents begin to teach children strategies of self-control, particularly at this very tender age? Well, we saw above that during this second year of life, we may hear children rehearsing instructions which have been given them by their parents, 'Not jump on bed', or 'Eat it all up'. Towards the end of the second year, we can hear toddlers instructing themselves in how to behave: 'Stroke the cat *gently*' and 'Put toys in box'. Clearly these are very early exercises in self-control and the children should be commended immediately (Box 3.7).

Box 3.7 Skills involving self-control which can be taught to toddlers in the second year

- To eat food with a suitable implement and not throw it on the floor.
- To brush teeth after breakfast and at the end of the day.
- To wait for a toy which another children is playing with – this will need plenty of training!
- To wait until Mum or carer has finished talking – not to interrupt.
- To wait for turns at the nursery or in the garden.
- To try to hold wee or poo until they can go into the toilet.

Another way of teaching self-control is by developing family rules, as discussed above. In one of my other books (Sutton 2006), and helped by a group of Family Support Workers in Luton with whom Di Hampton and I were developing training, I suggested some rules which, if followed more or less faithfully, could become a part of a little child's natural repertoire of self-control. For children of one to two years, they are as listed in Box 3.8.

Box 3.8 Sample rules for toddlers

- We hold hands when we're out and about.
- We sit at the table to eat and drink.
- We say 'Please', 'Thank you' and 'Sorry'.
- We put away toys when we've finished playing.
- We kiss, or blow a kiss, goodnight.
- No hitting or smacking in our family.
- No shouting or swearing in our house.

If these seem too idealistic or unattainable, we can ask families which *one* of the list they would like to identify as one goal for one week; we can then use coaching methods, say a text or a phone call to encourage progress towards, for example, 'We put away toys when we've finished playing'.

In the next chapter we shall consider how to promote wellbeing in children aged three to eight and their parents.

CHAPTER 4

Three to Eight Years

OVERVIEW

- Acknowledging risk factors
- Building on protective factors
- Encouraging the generous use of praise
- Encouraging authoritative parenting
- Developing family activities
- High quality early childhood education
- Supporting close home/nursery/school relationships
- Encouraging language and literacy
- Close supervision of the child
- Encouraging self-control by the child

ACKNOWLEDGING RISK FACTORS

There is extensive and irrefutable evidence that poverty has a major impact on educational outcomes for children. International studies demonstrate that children's educational achievement is one of the key areas affected by family incomes. As Ferguson, Bovaird and Mueller (2007), writing from a Canadian standpoint, highlight:

> Six poverty-related factors are known to impact child development in general and school readiness in particular:
> - the incidence of poverty
> - the depth of poverty
> - the duration of poverty

- ◦ the timing of poverty (e.g. the age of the child)
- ◦ community characteristics (e.g. concentration of poverty and crime in the neighbourhood, and school characteristics)
- ◦ the impact poverty has on the child's social network (parents, relatives and neighbours).

Ferguson and his team suggest that the evidence is 'clear and unanimous that poor children arrive at school at a cognitive and behavioural disadvantage'. Studies such as the Progress in International Reading Literacy Study (see NFER 2015) found a similar relationship between socioeconomic status and school achievement across the many countries in which data were gathered. It is not of course the direct impact of the amount of money coming into a household which has negative effects on children, but the way in which the low income increases parental stress, limits a healthy lifestyle and prevents access to community resources.

Parents who are greatly stressed are likely to have little patience with their young children. Yet there is overwhelming evidence that harsh parenting, involving shouting, bullying, rejection and aggression, is damaging to children (Mohr and Anderson 2002). Ever since Rutter, Giller and Hagell (1998) confirmed the association between hostile and critical parenting and antisocial behaviour, many other studies have confirmed this link, especially in the context of major neighbourhood disadvantage (e.g. Burnette *et al.* 2012).

Concerning inconsistency, a recent study by Scott *et al.* (2012) involving 278 families having children aged 4–7 in Inner London and a city in the south-west of England, where the children were at risk of poor social and academic outcomes, showed that harsh, inconsistent discipline was clearly associated with more severe child antisocial behaviour: the 25 per cent of parents using the most hostile discipline had children with twice the rate of serious behaviour problems. Mothers' depression and stress, as well as domestic violence, were additionally associated with child antisocial behaviour, while the symptoms of ADHD contributed to the child's difficulties. All these stressors, either separately or together, can be seen to increase the likelihood of children's experiencing disturbances in their development: some children may internalise their distress and become anxious or depressed in their turn; others may externalise their feelings and become hostile and aggressive.

This will not surprise us. A child who has an aggressive or abusive parent, whether father or mother, is likely to model his own behaviour on that of his parent; he will, as we all do, respond to perceived threat with one of the 'fight, flight, freeze' reactions (Box 4.1).

Box 4.1 Possible responses to perceived threat

- *Fight.* The child becomes angry and aggressive in his turn, rude or abusive to others. The angry feelings may escalate into violent behaviour.
- *Flight.* The child becomes fearful and withdrawn at home, and perhaps at playgroup and school.
- *Freeze.* The child becomes virtually immobile with fear, highly alert to possible further threats, hypervigilant and unable to trust others.

On the basis of extensive research, Scott and his team (2014, p.3) claim:

> Three factors that reliably predispose children to underachieve and become socially excluded in childhood with enduring effects into adulthood are (1) experiencing suboptimal parenting, such as lack of praise and encouragement, being subject to overly harsh, inconsistent discipline, (2) behaving disruptively and (3) being a poor reader.

As we have seen, the foundations of these difficulties are laid in the earliest years of life so that many children start formal education at age four or five having already experienced harshness, inconsistent discipline and lack of positive stimulation.

The issue of school readiness is particularly important in this period, three to eight years of age. We touched on this in Chapter 3, and we now explore the issue further. The authors of the most recent Ofsted report into good practice in school readiness, *Are you Ready? Good Practice in School Readiness* (Ofsted 2014), which focused on the age group 0–5, examined how the most successful early years providers achieved the objective of ensuring disadvantaged and vulnerable children are better prepared to start school. The inspectors report (p.4):

For too many children, especially those living in the most deprived areas, educational failure starts early. Gaps in achievement between the poorest children and their better-off counterparts are clearly established by the age of five. There are strong associations between a child's social background and their readiness for school as measured by their scores on entry into year 1. Too many children, especially those that are poor, lack a firm grounding in the key skills of communication, language, literacy and mathematics.

These authors continue:

Too many children start school without the range of skills they need. Across the country in 2013 only a half of all children reached a good level of development by the age of five (Department for Education 2013). For some children the picture was much worse. In over 50 local authorities less than a third of children reached this level... Too few who start school behind their peers catch up by the time they leave education.

The list of desirable abilities and skills which the inspectors see as requisite for children starting school is shown in Appendix 8. Michael Wilshaw, the Chief Inspector, believes that all parents should be provided with a list of these skills to help them to prepare their children.

In their report, the inspectors go on to note that vulnerable children need the very best provision, but that this is not reliably available. The most effective providers of early childhood education seem to identify very quickly the starting points of the children 'and use discrete adult-led sessions as part of a range of provision to accelerate progress.' Close links and partnerships between preschool and school settings were found to be particularly beneficial to the children, and particularly so if it was possible to engage parents as well.

BUILDING ON PROTECTIVE FACTORS

As will be apparent, the protective factors are frequently the counterpart of the risk factors: for example, supportive and confident parenting, the counterpart of rejecting and harsh parenting, is known to offer enormous benefits to young children, while warm and loving relationships protect them against rejection and blame. Such relationships have at least three separate positive impacts on children of this three to eight years age band.

First, they make emotional attachment between child and parent or caregiver stronger: as the child experiences, day by day, week by week, attentive, appreciative interactions with people who really care about him and his welfare, and as he comes to feel safe with them and to enjoy their company, so the emotional ties between him and his caregivers deepen; he becomes more closely attached to them. Second, as the child becomes more closely attached to his parents, so they respond to his wish to be with them and to interact with them by becoming ever more closely bonded with and protective of him; or, in everyday language, he comes to love them, and they come to love him. Third, as they commend him and his actions, his kindness, his care for other children or his willingness to be helpful, so the parents and caregivers are, whether they think of it in this way or not, rewarding and reinforcing his kind and helpful behaviour. These several interlocking processes, the increase in attachment and bonding and the reinforcement of desired behaviour, enhance and mutually strengthen each other.

ENCOURAGING THE GENEROUS USE OF PRAISE

So how can a helping person, professional or lay, be supportive in situations where parents are frantic with stress? First, of course, he or she has to be *perceived* by the child and family as 'helpful'. If such people are seen as busybodies, butting in where they are not wanted, they will not even get across the doorstep. But, assuming they are allowed into the house, then it will be essential to give time and space to the harassed parents and just to *listen* – to offer the empathic support which we know from abundant research can be invaluable. We explored this idea and the evidence of its importance in earlier chapters (see, for example, Table 1.1).

Let us work then from the point where the helper is accepted into the household and where, let us say, certain specific difficulties have been identified by the parent(s). These might arise from the stress experienced by a single mother, recently abandoned by her partner, as she cares for three children, aged five years, three years, and ten months. The loss of an adult member of the family and the financial support he was offering are likely to put extremely stressful pressures on her: just listening will be helpful. The helper must see the needs of the parent as paramount in this situation: unless the parent can cope, then the baby or child won't be able to. Parents matter. The helper may be able to guide the mother towards emergency resources or financial support to help her cope on a day-to-day basis. According to the boundaries of her role, the helper may be able to come to an arrangement to take one or two of the older children to Story Time at the local library once a week, so allowing the mother, desperate for sleep, to have an hour or two in bed while the baby naps and then get something on the table for tea.

Meanwhile the mother may be frantic about the specific behaviour of one of the children, say the three-year-old, who, upset by the departure of his daddy and distressed to see his mother so often in tears, will do nothing that he is asked, cheeks his mother and plagues the baby. His mother, who has previously had no problems with this child, is frantic with worry. She has tried everything – scolding him, depriving him of television, giving treats to the five-year-old but not to him – but still he will not do as he is told.

Let us turn to the principles of social learning theory which were introduced in Chapter 3. I remember visiting the mother of a tearaway three-year-old who was also coping with a small baby. After spending time getting to know this mother and her children during two visits, and listening empathically to her account of the stress her difficulties were causing her, I asked her if she had ever tried praising her little boy. She replied that there was nothing to praise him for: he was naughty, cheeky and aggressive – he was *never* good. I was able at this point to tell this mother briefly about the research I had done with over 40 families in Leicester and Leicestershire. In each family I had helped the parents, stressed and hassled as they were, to stop punishing their tearaway child for bad behaviour, *as this was in effect rewarding him for bad behaviour by giving him attention for it.* Instead I asked them whether there were any, very occasional, instances when the child *had* done as he was asked – had come when she called, had found a missing shoe, or had given a toy to the baby. There was always something which, with care, could be identified as 'good' behaviour by the tearaway child. This then, I explained, was the time when the mum should show, in some way, that she was pleased with him. However rarely this happened, she should at this point reward his positive behaviour with her praise and approval – in the language of psychology she should give him 'positive reinforcement'. The impact of this approval would make it more likely that it would happen again.

Once this mother had told me that she understood what I was suggesting, and once she had, with my encouragement, demonstrated that she could do what I was asking, I asked her to practise this approach until my visit the following week. She also agreed to keep a simple record of 'bad' and 'good' behaviour, putting a mark on a piece of paper or putting beans in a jar. For a week or so, no change was evident; in fact, *as the theory predicts*, the misbehaviour got worse. As the child realised that the strategies which he had used before to obtain his mum's attention were no longer working, so he increased the bad behaviour in an effort to regain this attention. With my explanations and support, however, this mother did not give up. Indeed, as the approach began to take effect and the record showed occasional good behaviour, she said she would try to find something every day which she could praise him for.

And so we went on… Towards the end of my contact with her, after about five or six weekly meetings, she met me delightedly one afternoon and reported the effects of praising her little son. She said:

- 'His behaviour is ten times better.
- His speech is coming on.
- He's interested in school work.
- He's happier.
- He's brilliant with the baby.
- He said to me, "I love you".
- Other people have noticed the change in him.
- The change is brilliant.'

All this had been achieved by this mother's switching her attention from her child's 'naughty' and negative behaviour to his 'good' and positive behaviour. *This principle underpins all the rigorously evaluated parenting programmes which address aggressive and disruptive behaviour by young children.* Other principles, such as spending a few minutes every day looking at a picture book or playing a simple game with each child (so-called 'nurture time' or 'special time'), are important as well, but attending to good behaviour is a fundamental plank of social learning theory.

A chart for recording instances of desired behaviour, such as a child's following an instruction when first asked, or of undesired behaviour, such as *not* following an instruction when first asked, is included as Appendix 9. This can be photocopied and used over several weeks. For my own experience of working with over 40 families in Leicester and Leicestershire who used this chart see my book *Helping Families with Troubled Children* (Sutton 2006).

Let's look in a bit more detail at why this approach has such positive effects. Figure 4.1 shows a cross section of the brain showing the 'reward pathways' and the amygdala which is associated with the detection of perceived threat.

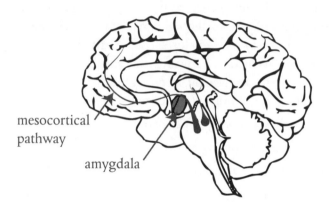

mesocortical
pathway

amygdala

Figure 4.1 Aspects of the reward and threat sensitive systems in the brain

Neurological underpinning of the reward and threat systems

Because safety and threat are so fundamental to survival, Nature has endowed us with brain systems which are acutely sensitive to these situations.

Events which are perceived as pleasurable and rewarding are mediated by brain systems marked by a dotted line in Figure 4.1; other events which are unpleasant and which are perceived as threatening or frightening are mediated by a brain network centred on the amygdala

(Zald 2003). So, if a parent commends a child, smiles at him and praises his behaviour, this is likely to be perceived as very rewarding by the child and he is likely to repeat the behaviour, for example coming when called. (It is noteworthy, however, that if a child has only heard rejecting and abusive terms, he may be completely disoriented by praise. Typically he will need individual, sensitive and tailored positive reinforcement to accustom him to encouragement and praise – perhaps by using dolls or puppets.)

If the child does not come when called and runs away when his mother wants him, she will, not surprisingly, shout at him and call him a bad boy, or worse. But if this is unpleasant, why does he repeat this behaviour? The explanation for this is the *rewarding impact of attention*. A child who receives very little positive or appreciative attention may find that misbehaving is one dependable way of getting him some attention, even if not of a pleasant kind. He is likely to go on misbehaving, *even if it brings him a smacking*, if that is the only form of attention he can get (see Box 3.3). Undesirable behaviour which is rewarded is likely to lead to more undesirable behaviour. Table 4.1 sets out some rewarding and unrewarding responses which parents and others can make to different patterns of behaviour by children in this age range of 3–8 years. Appendix 10a shows some appreciative remarks which parents can make to their child and Appendix 10b suggests some useful 'When…then…' phrases.

Table 4.1 Rewarding and penalising responses to children's behaviour

Rewards	Penalties
Cuddles, hugs and kisses	Being criticised, told off
Approving attention	Being ignored
Praise and admiration	Criticism and blame
Stickers on a chart	Time Out/Calm Down time
Simple outings, to a friend, to the park	Being taken straight home from an outing
Appreciative comments to grandparents, aunts and uncles, neighbours	Extra small chores
Allowed to stay up for an extra half hour	Being sent to bed early
Family outings, for example swimming	Loss of privileges

The necessity for occasional penalties

We have spent a good deal of time examining the importance of praise and positive feedback for young children, and this is indeed a key principle for bringing up happy children. However, it is sometimes necessary to impose a 'penalty' – a less harsh word than 'punishment' and one which will be familiar to many children because of its frequent use in the context of football. Among the list of penalties shown in Table 4.1 is the practice of 'Time Out', for which some practitioners have substituted the term 'Calm Down time' – the meaning of which is indeed much clearer. Whatever the practice is called, if after being warned a child continues with misbehaviour, be it rudeness, aggressiveness, not following an instruction or wilfully doing the opposite of what the parent requested, then he or she should be sent to a designated place for them to calm down.

Evidence from my own research

As explained above, in my own research (Sutton 2001) I helped parents to withdraw their attention from irritating and difficult behaviour, such as the child pestering, teasing and not doing what they were asked to do, and instead to attend to the few occasions when the child played calmly, was helpful to a brother or sister, or did comply with what they were asked to do. Gradually, some wonderful changes took place. Within three to four weeks, parents reported that their difficult child had become not only easier to manage, but had become more loving. One mother, who had despaired of her child's behaviour, said, 'He is more affectionate, loving. He left a message saying, "I love you Mum". People have noticed a difference. Two people have said what a difference in him.' Another said, 'He comes and gives me a love. I like that, he never did that before. The difference in him is unbelievable. People say, "What's the matter with L?" thinking he is ill. The teacher said he is a different child, he will sit down and listen to a story.' A third said, 'He is more affectionate. He seems to be happier in himself. Other people have commented on how much calmer he is. We were beginning to feel such failures…'

As I wrote when reporting these data: 'It is particularly noteworthy that in five of the six reports, the mother reported that other people, not just the mother herself, have commented on the improvement in the child's behaviour. This addresses the commonly voiced criticism of parent management training that because everyone is calmer following the training, we are dealing simply with *a change in the mother's perception of the child's behaviour*, rather than an actual change (Sutton 2001).

This was delightful work to do: to share with parents their joy that a child who had seemed alienated from them, whom they didn't know how to control, was once again biddable, helpful and, above all, lovable, was intensely rewarding to me. Since then, teaching and disseminating this body of knowledge in all ways possible has become my life's work.

ENCOURAGING AUTHORITATIVE PARENTING

As we saw in Chapter 3, authoritative parents tend to be high in both warmth and control (Box 4.2).

Box 4.2 Characteristic behaviours of authoritative parents

Authoritative parents:

- are affectionate and nurturing to their children
- praise behaviour they approve of and would like to see more of
- set clear limits for behaviour
- make clear how they would like their child to behave
- respond to the child's needs, for example for comfort and attention
- spend time with their children and talk to them about shared interests
- are unlikely to use physical punishment
- may use 'Time Out' to discipline misbehaving children.

We have already discussed warm and appreciative parenting in some detail above, so let us now turn to other aspects of authoritative parenting.

Giving a clear and firm instruction

Helpers can enable parents to become more authoritative by coaching them in speaking firmly to a young child. This can be done very successfully by role-play. The instruction should be brief, clear and refer to one task only: for example, 'Tommy, come downstairs *now* please', as distinct from, 'We've got to go out so come and have your tea and bring Teddy from the floor in my bedroom.' A young child will lose the last parts of the message.

In much of my work with parents the mum and I would find a time when the child was at nursery or asleep; I would role-play the child while she would be herself. We would plan a little exercise: she would tell me, as Tommy, 'her child', that in a short time I must stop playing with the blocks or crayons, as we have, say, to go and fetch an older brother from school. After this warning, a minute or two later she would follow it with an instruction to come so that she could help me put on my coat.

At first parents often got very embarrassed when practising like this, but we would soon get into the way of it. Typically the mother would speak very gently at first; I would ignore her completely and go on with what I was doing. She would repeat the instruction a little more firmly, but often in a pleading way: again I would ignore her. After several goes, when I, as Tommy, took not the slightest notice of her I would come out of role and say that she would need to get my attention, if necessary go up to me, crouch down, look into my eyes and give her instruction much more firmly. Some mothers would find this difficult, but I would confirm that Tommy needed a very clear message – and we would have another go. Eventually I would be able to say to her, 'Right, I now feel you mean what you say!' and I would mentally put the crayons aside.

At other times we would carry out the role-play over the phone. With parents whom I had never met, but who had entered my research study, I was able to help them achieve a really firm tone of voice with five or six run-throughs; more important, they would subsequently tell me they had been able to put this new skill of giving a clear instruction into practice and that the child was beginning to comply. We laughed a lot during this telephone coaching; it was really fun to do.

Principles for practice in using Time Out/Calm Down time

Sometimes, despite our best efforts, children pay no attention to our instructions and insist on behaving in ways which are completely unacceptable: hitting and kicking other children or even their parents, rudeness to adults inside or outside the home, deliberately ignoring instructions, taking other people's possessions or breaking household items just for the sake of doing so. In these circumstances, it has been found that the simplest and most effective response by the caregivers is to give one warning and then if there is no compliance to place the child in the Time Out or Calm Down place. *The essence of the experience for the child is that he or she is ignored, so that they do not receive the reward of attention.* Box 4.3 sets out some of the key principles involved.

Box 4.3 Principles for using Time Out or Calm Down time (Sutton and Hampton 2013)

1. Never use a frightening place for Time Out, but do use a place which is safe, unrewarding and dull: the foot of the stairs, standing or sitting in a corner facing the wall, an empty room, a hallway.

2. Always check for safety.

3. Never threaten Time Out and fail to follow through: give one warning only.

4. You must be consistent. The child cannot learn the rules about how you want him or her to behave unless you are consistent.

5. Never lock a child in a room. Just keep returning him or her to the Time Out place, for a short period of time, insisting that he stays until he realises that you really mean it. Keep as calm as you possibly can.

6. Do not talk to the child while he is in Time Out.

---

7. A useful rule of thumb for how long a child should remain in Time Out is the number of minutes corresponding to the child's age. For example:

    - a two-year-old remains two minutes on each occasion
    - a five-year-old remains five minutes on each occasion
    - a ten-year-old remains 10 minutes on each occasion.

8. A kitchen timer is very useful here. Explain to the child to listen for the ring.

9. If a young child will not stay in the Time Out place, such as at the foot of the stairs, sit behind him, one step above, and hold his shoulders firmly.

10. There is no point in making the Time Out interval very long. We are trying to help the child learn a new association between misbehaving and the inevitability of the penalty. He will learn this better from each instance of misbehaving being followed every single time by a brief Time Out than from misbehaving being followed occasionally by Time Out for an arbitrary period of time.

11. If the child who has been placed in Time Out repeats the same misbehaviour as soon as he comes out of Time Out, then return him to the Time Out place immediately. If need be, repeat this several times each day, so that an association is learned.

12. Whoever put the child in Time Out takes him out. Then find something which you can praise or commend him for. Remember the '5 praises a day' principle.

13. Do persevere! Carry on as suggested even if you feel hopeless.

14. Keep a simple record of how often you use Time Out each day. If you are consistent it will probably show first an increase over several days and then a decrease.

15. *Things may get worse before they get better!* The child will work hard to keep his dominant position. But the message will get through if you persevere firmly and calmly: you are in charge now.

If items appear at home which do not belong to the children

It is very common for children of this age group to pick up things in shops or in the houses of their friends which do not belong to them. This may in part be as a result of the child not understanding that things in shops have to be paid for – and what a difficult thing this is to understand for a young child! All these marvellous items are spread out in front of them and they see other people picking them up and putting them in a basket or trolley, but they have to learn that they may not do the same. Why on earth not!? In some settings such as playgroups or nursery schools they may be allowed to help themselves to toys or play materials, but in others they may not. I am shocked by the way in which some shops still deliberately display sweets and other attractive items at the very levels where young children will see them and demand them.

But another reason why things arrive home from school or from other children's houses is that the child may be seeking comfort by pocketing items which he does know belong in the shop or to his friend. I have coined the term 'comfort stealing' for this activity, and am glad that the term is gaining acceptance. In Box 4.4 I offer some suggestions for dealing with this. I have to acknowledge that I have been unable to find reference to randomised controlled trials to underpin these suggestions, but since the principles are closely in line with principles of social learning theory and since I employed them successfully when seeking to help parents who had sewn up the pockets of their little daughter's clothes whenever she visited the house of a friend, I offer them with a good deal of confidence.

Box 4.4 Responding to 'comfort stealing'

1. When the 'stealing' is discovered, make it very clear that taking things which do not belong to us is unacceptable.

2. The aim is to be very clear with the child, but not to act utterly shocked by her behaviour. (I heard recently of a small child who was taken to the police station where the parent requested that a policeman should tell her very strongly that she must not take things which were not hers.)

3. If possible, put things right. For example, pencils and rubbers should be returned to school, perhaps via an understanding teacher. Some schools have 'amnesty days' when items taken home can be tactfully returned by parents with no questions asked.

4. If the items have come home from a friend's house, explain calmly to the child as soon as possible that she should not have brought the toy home from Jane's house and it must go back. Say you are going to contact Jane's mummy and explain calmly that a toy has come home from her house and will be going back. Keep the whole thing low-key.

5. Consider the possibility that this behaviour may be 'comfort stealing' – a bit like 'comfort eating', when grown-ups nibble food we do not need. What might the child need comforting for?

6. Try to make sure the child receives some extra comfort; for example time spent with her, playing, chatting, looking at stories and so on. *Time spent with the child rather than giving presents is what matters.*

7. Switch attention towards 'rewarding trustworthy behaviour'. Find little occasions when the child can be helped to demonstrate trustworthiness: delivering a message, posting a letter in a box while a parent is nearby, buying a small item while the parent waits nearby, bringing the right change from a small purchase.

8. Then commend her for her trustworthy behaviour. Continue gently to reinforce this behaviour over time and mention to Auntie and Grandpa that you can trust her to complete small tasks and to carry out promises.

9. Demonstrate trustworthiness in your own behaviour. Always keep promises and don't promise anything you can't be sure of keeping. Say things like 'We'll see...' rather than promising 'We'll buy you a new dress...' if you are not sure you can afford it.

DEVELOPING FAMILY ACTIVITIES

There are plenty of low-key games and activities which a helper can introduce to families with children in this age group. They can bring pleasure to all members, not just the children. Above all, they help parents to enjoy time spent with their children and to have fun together as a family.

A range of family activities

These can be cost-free, not too messy, but valuable as enriching family life and including everyone. It may need the helper to introduce the games and activities but as everyone gets to learn how to take part, he or she can play a less central role and support the parents in initiating the games themselves. Box 4.5 gives a few simple but enjoyable activities which everyone can play according to their ages.

Useful family rules or guidelines

An important step in helping families can be to work out family or house rules. Children of all ages can make suggestions, which the whole family then discuss for their suitability and practicality. Mum or Dad acts as chairperson. Box 4.6 gives some suggestions.

Box 4.5 Simple games and songs for all the family

- *I spy:* 'I spy with my little eye, something beginning with B.' Book? No. Baby? No. Ball? Yes!
- *Simple card games:* Snap and Sevens.
- *Matching pairs of cards:* Pairs of domino cards are turned face down and spread out over the table or floor. Players take turns to try to remember where they are placed. If correct, they take the pair and have another go. If incorrect, they put the cards back where they were, face down, and it is the next person's turn. The winner is the person with the most pairs, but the winning is *not* important: it's the fun of playing and trying to remember positions.
- *Reciting nursery rhymes*, with actions.
- *Jigsaws*, with everyone helping.
- *Hunt the thimble*, or equivalent, such as an apple or carrot.
- *Singing together* – anything, and *everyone* is encouraged to sing, without criticism. Everyone sits in a circle, children on the ground, and simple songs, like 'The wheels on the bus' or 'Row, row, row your boat…' are sung again and again. Everyone claps to the rhythm. Below is a version which we have written which is sung to the same tune. We hope it will be sung in playgroups and Children's Centres and that the children will sing it there and at home, so that parents get the message!

Praise, praise, praise your child,

At least 5 times a day.

'Good girl!', 'Good boy!' and 'I love you',

Those are things to say!'

> **Box 4.6 Sample family guidelines for children of three to eight years (Sutton 2006)**
>
> - We say nice things to each other.
> - We help each other.
> - We listen to each other at meal times.
> - TV off during meal times.
> - Evening meal together – at the table if possible.
> - Up and dressed in time for breakfast.
> - School clothes and school bag prepared the night before.
> - When accidents happen, tell a grown-up truthfully.
> - No secrets from parents (surprises are all right).

Everyone then tries to follow the rules – in a light-hearted way. Anyone who is successful in, say, getting up in time, gets a family clap; if they are unsuccessful, Mum says, 'OK, try again tomorrow!' Children encourage the parents to follow the rules, but again, in a light-hearted way. Sometimes, say at a meal, everyone can practise saying something kind about everyone else. Mum might say, 'Thank you Danny for finding my keys.' Danny might say, 'I liked it when Jack shared his chocolate with me.' Lucy might say, 'Jill looked at a story book with me.' And Jill might say, 'I was pleased when Grandma fetched me from school.' Mum and Dad, too, can take part. Mum might get a clap for clearing out the fridge and Dad for cleaning the car. These examples may sound a bit 'cheesy' but they all deserve a clap; they model the giving of positive messages to children about each other, and they give positive reinforcement for desirable patterns of behaviour.

Doing physical activities together

Box 4.7 gives a list of suggestions by Ken Fox, of Bristol University.

Box 4.7 Ways to get active with your kids (NHS)

1. Walk or cycle with the children to playgroup or school as often as possible.

2. Build a den with them in the school holidays; or, under supervision, encourage them to climb a tree.

3. Go roller skating or skateboarding indoors or out. Children love to have parents watch them or, even better, show parents how to learn these skills.

4. Do an activity challenge together, such as a fun run or a walk for charity.

5. Take a dog for a walk. If you don't have one, ask to borrow a friend's or a neighbour's dog.

6. Support children in sports clubs or other physical activities. Beavers and Rainbows include physical items on their programmes.

7. Every weekend try to do something active with the children: take them to the swings, slides and climbing frames as a regular destination with Frisbee or football to follow.

8. Encourage the whole family to learn to swim, including all the adults. This is a lifelong investment of time and money and may contribute to saving lives.

9. Fly a kite together.

10. Arrange a day at the beach together.

Adapted from Professor Ken Fox's NHS activity tips

If involvement in these activities can be accompanied by, say, a chart in which family members set goals for themselves about what they want to reach, such as 'Swim a width across the pool' and if these achievements can be noted with stars and 'texting to tell Grandma', the child's pleasure can be strengthened if Dad or Mum also get involved.

Helping parents get a bit of time to themselves

This was one wish which many mothers told me about: the chance to have just a few minutes, say ten or fifteen, to themselves, to look at the paper, to have a quiet cup of coffee or just to put their feet up without being pestered by a child. Using social learning theory, we were able to achieve this with this age group of children quite smoothly. Box 4.8 shows an example of how this might be done.

Box 4.8 How parents can get a bit of time to themselves

- Get the child's full attention and then explain that Mum/Dad needs a short rest and they are going to sit on the sofa with a cup of tea or coffee (or whatever).

- Mum is not to be interrupted during this time, so if the child comes to talk to her she will not talk to him; she will not even look at him.

- Put out a toy that the child hasn't played with for, say, a week or two. (This means that some toys will need putting away every so often so that they can be produced again as near-novelties.) Drawings and colouring are always popular.

- If he keeps on making demands or talking to her, she will not reply, and will not even look at him. She will drink her coffee, read the paper, and rest her feet for those ten or fifteen minutes.

- If he lets her rest, however, at the end of that time she will look at pictures with him, will read him a story, play Snap or have 10 or 15 minutes of happy time together which he can choose.

- If he does not let her rest but keeps pestering, she will not spend time with him.

- But she will try again tomorrow.

With just a few hiccups, this strategy was frequently successful and could be used at least twice a day, say once in the morning and once in the afternoon, to give harassed parents a few minutes to themselves.

Time spent with a parent or relative is one of the simplest of rewards, and is often enjoyed by both child and adult, especially if it involves looking at a book together, playing a game or doing a jigsaw.

HIGH QUALITY EARLY CHILDHOOD EDUCATION

In this area, there is a wealth of excellent research. The Effective Provision of Pre-School Education (EPPE) Project (Sylva *et al.* 2004) is a European longitudinal study of young children's development between the ages of three and seven. It examined background characteristics of the children's parents and home environments and the preschool settings where children attended. These included local authority and private nurseries, playgroups, nursery schools and nursery classes. Some key findings are summarised in Box 4.9.

Box 4.9 Impact of attending a preschool

- Preschool experience, compared with none, enhances all-round development in children.

- Length of attendance (in months) is important: an earlier start (under age three years) is related to better intellectual development.

- Full-time attendance leads to no better gains for children than part-time attendance.

- Disadvantaged children benefit significantly from good quality preschool experiences, especially where they are with a mixture of children from different social backgrounds.

- Overall, disadvantaged children tend to attend preschool for shorter periods of time than those from more advantaged groups (around 4–6 months less).

- There are significant differences between individual preschool settings and their impact on children. Some settings are more effective than others in promoting positive child outcomes.

- Good quality can be found across all types of early years settings; however, quality is higher overall in settings integrating care and education and in nursery schools.

Effects of quality and specific practices in preschool

In addition, the researchers identified specific characteristics of staff and practices which enhanced the children's experience (Box 4.10).

Box 4.10 Characteristics of preschool which enhance children's development

- High quality preschooling is related to better intellectual and social/behavioural development for children.

- Settings that have staff with higher qualifications have higher quality scores and the children make more progress.

- Quality indicators include warm interactive relationships with children, having a trained teacher as manager and a good proportion of trained teachers on the staff.

- Where settings view educational and social development as complementary and equal in importance, children make better all-round progress.

- Effective pedagogy includes interactions traditionally associated with the term 'teaching', the provision of instructive learning environments and 'sustained shared thinking' to extend children's learning.

The importance of learning at home

The researchers also examined the contribution which can be made to children's development and wellbeing via learning at home, and they reported (Sylva *et al.* 2004, p.5):

> The home learning environment was only moderately associated with parents' educational or occupational level and was more strongly associated with children's intellectual and social development than either parental education or occupation. *In other words what parents do with their children is more important than who parents are.'* (my italics).

This does not mean that parents have actively to teach their children at home in formal ways, but that it is very beneficial to children if those who care for them can *talk* informally about all the day-to-day things that they see about them at home. It is helpful, for example, if those who care for children talk, at meal times, about where bread, milk and apples come from – while in the world outside, cars, dogs, trees, clouds and men mending the road are always interesting. Appendix 11 is a simple cartoon with a kiddie asking, *'Please Talk to ME!'* While so many parents understandably find support and friendship by means of their smartphones and other equipment, they may not realise what wonderful opportunities for stimulating their children's imagination and vocabulary they have just by talking to them and sharing with them the wonders of the world.

Helping children who need extra support before starting school

The Ofsted inspectors who recently published the results of their investigations of facilities for preschool children noted that vulnerable children need the very best provision, but that this is not reliably available. We saw above that the most effective providers of early childhood education seem to identify very quickly the starting points of the children and that close links and partnerships between preschool and school settings were found to be particularly beneficial to the children, *and particularly so if it was possible to engage parents as educators as well.*

It is obviously constructive if the helper, professional or lay, knows which skills the Ofsted inspectors have pinpointed as necessary for a child to be ready for school (see Appendix 8). Many parents may not know what will be expected of their child, but helpers may be in a position to explore the list with parents and to see if there are any specific skills they can all practise together with the child. If the items on the list can be 'ticked off' one by one as the child acquires them, there will be grounds for everyone to clap each other, to practise the skill again and again and to demonstrate it to Aunty Betty or Grandma.

SUPPORTING CLOSE HOME/NURSERY/ SCHOOL RELATIONSHIPS

It is clearly beneficial if parents and school staff can work together to enable young children to acquire and develop the key skills asked for by the Ofsted inspectors: these abilities can best be achieved if they are modelled and taught in nursery and in preschool settings and if parents are shown how to prepare their children to practise them in school. It follows that it is helpful to all concerned if a warm bond exists or can be developed between parents and nursery nurses or other staff and, later, with the child's teachers.

It is increasingly the practice for teachers and staff in nursery schools actively to develop close links with the parents of young children in their localities – with very encouraging outcomes. For example, in Luton, teachers and other staff believed that improved home–school liaison was a priority objective and they identified four targets:

1.   To build up the confidence of parents.

2.   To improve parenting skills.

3.   To enable parents to support their children at home.

4.   To encourage parents to take a more active part in school life.

Box 4.11 expands on these targets.

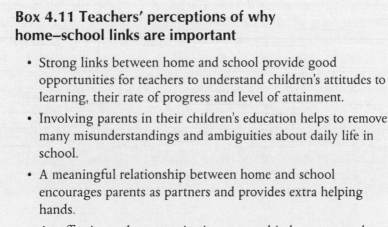

Box 4.11 Teachers' perceptions of why home–school links are important

- Strong links between home and school provide good opportunities for teachers to understand children's attitudes to learning, their rate of progress and level of attainment.
- Involving parents in their children's education helps to remove many misunderstandings and ambiguities about daily life in school.
- A meaningful relationship between home and school encourages parents as partners and provides extra helping hands.
- An effective and communicative partnership between teachers and parents establishes an environment where children have a sense of security, familiarity and cultural freedom which, in turn, enhances learning.

In this particular school, the vehicle for building close home–school links was 'sustainable development' so, over time, parents were initially invited to take part and then involved in improving the rather stark school building and its environment. The then headteacher reported:

'Both inside and outside our school we have plants in every nook and cranny. A small courtyard provides an attractive central "green" area and even the car park is edged with plant troughs and climbing plants. Either myself or the Deputy Headteacher is present on the playground from 8.50a.m. to greet and talk to parents.'

She describes other developments:

'We have adapted a spare classroom to use as a Parents' Room and have tried to make it homely… We hold a meeting of the Parents' Club once a fortnight and the programme of activities includes consultations when we ask parents for their views. There are also opportunities for parents to share their expertise with others, for example on behaviour management, as well as workshop and information-giving sessions led by school staff and other agencies.

'We hold several social events each year such as the Christmas and Eid parent/teacher parties, Harvest Brunch and the Autumn and Summer School Fairs where parents and staff have opportunities to get to know each other. In our particular school differences of language often prove to be a barrier to good communication. Administrative and teaching staff with community languages are available every morning from 8.45a.m. and after school. Many parents are keen to learn English and consequently language classes are held four afternoons a week.

'Children's education does not finish when they leave school at the end of the day. If we want parents to become real partners in the education of their children, then we must be prepared to spend time and effort in helping them to acquire the skills and knowledge needed to help their children at home.'

ENCOURAGING LANGUAGE AND LITERACY

We saw in the first section of this chapter that three factors reliably predispose children to underachieve and become socially excluded in childhood: experiencing suboptimal or ineffective parenting, behaving disruptively and being a poor reader. A study of particular interest in this field is that of Beckett *et al.* (2012), which is part of the Helping Children Achieve series of investigations. The study involved 215 children aged 5–7 from a disadvantaged inner London borough and from a city in the south-west of England who met criteria for displaying disruptive behaviour. They were randomly allocated to one of the four following conditions:

- a programme to improve behaviour and relationships (the Incredible Years – IY)
- a programme to improve literacy (Supporting Parents on Kids Education in Schools – SPOKES)
- both programmes combined
- a telephone helpline – control condition.

Immediately after the programmes all parents reported that they felt more confident in dealing with their child, that disruptive behaviour had diminished and that reading had improved, compared with the control group. Nine to eleven months after the start of the programme, interviews confirmed a reduction in disruptive behaviour for all three interventions compared with the control group. However, the startling finding was that literacy tests showed that children who had attended the IY group had made a clear gain in reading but no such gain was evident for children whose parents were allocated to the SPOKES literacy programme. The researchers explored the notion that it was the increase in positive parenting (encouragement and praise) and the reduction in negative parenting (criticism and inconsistent discipline) which had contributed to improvements not only in relationships and behaviour but also in improved reading.

A popular and effective approach in helping children to learn to read has been Shared Reading. With this method, the teacher, parent or other helper uses a very large book with very large text, visible to children sitting at the back of a semicircle, and goes through the story on several consecutive days with different objectives for different days:

Day 1 – The focus is on the story, for example, *The Gruffalo*.

Day 2 – The focus is on the characters in the story.

Day 3 – The focus is on the meaning of punctuation marks.

Day 4 – The focus is on the voices of the characters.

Day 5 – The focus is on the outcome of the story.

Examples of this can be seen on YouTube [8]Advantages of the method, which appear to contribute to greater improvements than the 'reading in turn' method are:

- It provides struggling readers with group and teacher support.
- Familiarity with the text provides sight word knowledge and fluency.
- Pupils can enjoy text that they may not be able to read on their own.
- All children enjoy success together.

If this approach can be shared with parents, so that they and their children learn together, what advantages can accrue over several generations!

CLOSE SUPERVISION OF THE CHILD

This is the age range when families are continuing or are putting in place habits which will serve them ill or well in the future. A paper of great importance by Odgers *et al.* (2012) updates findings from the British Environmental Risk (E-Risk) Longitudinal Twin Study, involving 2232 children. This team has reported a graded relationship between neighbourhood socioeconomic status (SES) and children's antisocial behaviour which:

- can be observed at school entry
- widens across childhood
- remains after controlling for family-level SES and risk, *but which,*
- is completely mediated by maternal warmth and parental monitoring (defined throughout as supportive parenting). In other words, the risks to the children can be completely offset by the emotional warmth of the mother towards her child and the extent of supervision of the growing child by the parents.

---

8   See, for example, *Primary Shared Reading*, www.youtube.com/ watch?v=5Vlg1cp5PVk.

Thus, although there were measurable effects of socioeconomic status on children's antisocial behaviour as early as age five, these were completely offset by 'two supportive parenting practices defined here as maternal warmth and parental monitoring'.

We have discussed maternal warmth at length in previous chapters, and authoritative parenting continues to be of great importance throughout childhood. However, as children move into the primary school age, the second key principle, monitoring children's whereabouts, becomes of great importance. The habit of being absolutely certain where one's children are, whom they are with, what time they are due back and who will be bringing them back should be firmly in place, and practised until they leave home as adults! Yet it is exceedingly difficult to impose rules of letting parents know where they are and of being firm about coming-in times when children are rising adolescents: it is never easy, but it is easier if the practice has been in place for years, indeed ever since they were old enough to go to school. We shall return to this principle in the next chapter, concerning children of 9 to 13 years.

ENCOURAGING SELF-CONTROL BY THE CHILD

We saw in Chapter 3 that all sorts of positive features are associated with helping children to develop self-control – in essence to practise responsibility for themselves and towards others. It is during this period, three to eight years of age, that patterns of socialisation introduced to the child from without, that is, external socialisation, are often internalised by the child. For example, habits of eating, drinking, washing, brushing teeth, reading, playing sport, activities that are routinely practised within the family, become part of the child's habits – for good or ill. If parents can encourage children during this period to take on certain small responsibilities – to feed pets and to see that their cages are clean, to put dirty clothes into the washing machine, and to check that items needed the next day for school are put into school bags the night before – these habits will become part of the child's routines probably for the rest of his life.

Pocket money

The same applies to the giving, spending and saving of pocket money. Although the research does not seem to have been published in a recognised academic journal, a study in this field involving 12,000 parents across Europe suggests that many parents typically begin giving pocket money to children from about the age of four. The middle amount of pocket money given weekly to British children under five is about £2.00. It is not stated what items had to be purchased from this sum. A researcher in this study (Boyce 2014) stated: 'Our research suggests a correlation between adults who were given pocket money as a child and their ability to better manage their finances later in life. Allowing children some element of financial control may be one way to help them realise the value of money and build basic budgeting skills, which will help prepare them for financial independence when they leave home.'

Here is a field, then, in which with parents' help children can begin to develop self-control in a limited but very important area: financial self-management. Box 4.12 indicates some of the advantages of giving pocket money.

Box 4.12 Advantages of giving pocket money to children aged 4–8

1. It allows self-determination and independence, but under the oversight of the parents.

2. Once the pocket money is spent, it is spent.

3. Children can learn the principle of saving up for items they want.

4. They can learn to go to a post office or bank and see their savings accumulate.

5. They learn the principle of [modest] interest on savings.

In this chapter, then, we have considered some of the major developments occurring in the lives of children of around three to eight years. In the next chapter we shall examine the years from nine to 13, as children move away from childhood and become 'young people'.

CHAPTER 5

Nine to Thirteen Years

OVERVIEW

- Acknowledging risk factors
- Building on protective factors
- Encouraging authoritative parenting
- The importance of fathers
- Parents' involvement in children's activities
- Close supervision of the young person's whereabouts
- Parenting/child management skills training
- Devising written agreements
- A strong school ethos: backing school standards
- Mentoring programmes
- Multisystemic therapy
- Using cognitive behavioural principles in work with parents
- Other approaches with a strong evidence base

This period in a child's life encompasses many major transitions: he or she develops physically and physiologically, typically moves from primary to secondary education, may assume greater responsibilities at home or at school and often matures into wider relationships within the community. As before, we shall briefly examine risk factors for children during this period and then go on to focus on the protective factors and ones which can enhance a child's passage into adolescence and adulthood.

ACKNOWLEDGING RISK FACTORS

The same risk factors, particularly social deprivation and disadvantage which were powerful prejudicial factors during earlier periods of a child's life, continue to be powerful influences during this period. For, as we have emphasised, children are the victims of the *cumulative risks*, both those which have impacted upon their lives in earlier years and those currently affecting them: mothers and fathers who may themselves have mental health difficulties are often coping with low incomes and poor accommodation; their children may have insecure attachments and may attend schools with overstretched teachers, leading to the children's low achievement. All these factors interact and contribute to prejudicing the children's future.

In addition to challenges in gaining skills in communication and literacy, rejection by their peers is a further hazard which children who are beginning to display patterns of aggressive behaviour during the final years of primary school are likely to encounter – and they are very likely to take those patterns with them into secondary school. For example, Lane *et al.* (2004) report: 'Peer rejection often leads to children joining deviant peer groups which provide further training in deviant behaviour and increases the risk of drug abuse and antisocial behaviour… (Taylor and Biglan 1998)'.

Parental supervision is of the greatest importance at this stage. By the age of nine or ten, some children begin to report that their peers are of similar or greater importance to them than their parents (Reid and Patterson 1989). Yet as children seek to spend more time with their friends, some parents seem to reduce rather than increase their supervision of their children. As Berk (2006, p.511) summarises:

> Unfortunately, children from conflict-ridden homes who already display serious antisocial tendencies are most likely to experience inadequate parental monitoring. As a result, few if any limits are placed on out-of-home activities and association with antisocial friends, who encourage their hostile style of responding.

Earlier, seminal studies by Wilson (1980, 1987) compared the rates of offending of children living in the inner city or the suburbs according to whether the level of parental control exercised by the parents was 'strict', 'intermediate' or 'lax'. She found that in inner city neighbourhoods the offending rate of boys from 'lax' families was over two and a half times that of those from 'strict' families. Subsequently, Farrington and Coid (2003) confirmed that lax supervision of a child was an important risk factor for both chronic offending and antisocial personality in adulthood. Moreover, we saw above (Odgers *et al.* 2012) that firm supervision, together with maternal warmth, were the two key variables which distinguished children at serious risk of becoming offenders from those at less risk.

Truancy is a very likely outcome if a child is unsettled in school with few friends, unable to keep up with other pupils and repeatedly failing. Such a child may also be unhappy at home. So why should he continue to put himself through these horrible experiences? Much easier to stay away. The school environment, including how school staff respond to the truancy, plays a critical role in its management. We shall consider positive responses below.

The onset of puberty, with its accompanying physical and psychological developments, is likely to be a time of self-consciousness and embarrassment among both boys and girls. It is helpful to think of the stresses occurring at around this time as follows:

- Physical and physiological changes
- Emotional changes
- Concern about identity – sexual, cultural and religious
- Relationships with the peer group
- Interpersonal tensions, especially with parents and family members.

The physical changes of puberty are marked, with the peak growth spurt in girls occurring at around 11 years and at around 14 years in boys, so that girls of the same age in the same class at school can appear as young women alongside little boys. Growth spurts are of course accompanied by other physiological changes, such as primary and secondary sexual developments, all of which can lead to an increase in self-consciousness in young people. Alongside these changes may come a preoccupation with identity and perhaps an urge to abandon conventions observed by parents such as how to dress, how to spend one's time and how to choose friends: arguments with family members and school authority figures are common.

BUILDING ON PROTECTIVE FACTORS

It would be a mistake to assume that children will inevitably experience major difficulties as they move towards and into adolescence. As Coleman and Hendry (2000, p.94) report:

> In spite of a general public belief that adolescence is characterised by high levels of conflict in the home, research does not support this conclusion. While there are many issues about which parents and young people disagree in general, relationships appear more positive than negative. Many factors will have an impact on the level of conflict and, in particular, good communication between parents and young people has the effect of reducing conflict. As might be expected, conflict is highest where parents themselves have poor relationships, where the family is experiencing stress because of environmental factors, and where there is a longstanding impairment of parental function.

If families have been able to provide a home to which children and young people can return, confident of their welcome and supported by firm guidelines about behaviour towards each other and other people, many of them pass through this stage without great problems. So what can practitioners and other helpers do to help maintain this equilibrium?

ENCOURAGING AUTHORITATIVE PARENTING

As was found in relation to children in younger age ranges, confident and authoritative parenting confers many advantages upon children: the expression of warmth and love to children by parents with firm boundaries set and enforced, with clear expectations about behaviour and time spent together in enjoyable activities – all these lay the foundations for high self-esteem among the children and acceptance by the community. These same circumstances, carried into the teenage years, become all the more important as young people test the boundaries and challenge parental guidelines. I remember well a student telling us how in her family the grandmother had admonished the children as they prepared to go to secondary school or to college: 'You are to remember that you belong to the James family. We have a good name and we expect you to maintain it.' The student said that these clear expectations had influenced her decisions as she grew up and entered the adult world: would grandmother see her intended actions as upholding or diminishing the reputation of the James family?

The principles of social learning theory which were set out in earlier chapters are absolutely as valid for this age group as for younger children. Primary and secondary school children benefit from hearing that their parents love them and care about their behaviour just as much as do children at primary school – although they may not wish to have this spoken about in the company of their friends. I remember visiting a family in which a youngster was beginning to kick over the traces and talking to the mother about her son: 'I think the world of our Jack,' she said, 'but I'd never let him know it...' When I asked why she wouldn't let him know it, she said that it would make him big-headed. I was able to tell her that there wasn't much danger of this and that children really benefit from hearing their parents say appreciative things to them and that sincere, warm praise could only be beneficial. One of the health visitors with whom I was discussing this reluctance many people appear to have to say positive things to each other, and especially to children, commented, 'Yes, we're a bit stiff in England, aren't we?' Well yes, I think we are and I am doing my best in this book to soften that stiffness!

THE IMPORTANCE OF FATHERS

There seems still to be a great shortage of rigorous research on the significance of fathers within families and the relationships between them and their families in the Western world – particularly concerning them and their adolescent children. However, in a systematic review of longitudinal studies of the impact of fathers' involvement in their children's developmental outcomes, Sarkadi et al. (2008, p.157) report:

> It would seem that active and regular engagement in the child [by the father] predicts a range of positive outcomes... Father engagement reduces the frequency of behavioural problems in boys and psychological problems in young women; it also enhances cognitive development while decreasing criminality and economic disadvantage in low SES families.

Opportunities for a child to identify with his or her father, his values and interests, the chance to acquire the father's knowledge and skills in, say, sport, technology, music or in the creative arts, as well as to feel the security of a person committed to his or her welfare – these must all be of enduring support to a growing young person. If parents and aunts, uncles, cousins and grandparents also form part of the child's family system so that he or she is supplied with a rich and enduring network of relationships all concerned for the young person's welfare, this can support them in later adolescence and adulthood. The saying, 'It takes a village to raise a child' is founded on great wisdom.

PARENTS' INVOLVEMENT IN CHILDREN'S ACTIVITIES

Seeing one's parents taking part in sport, music-making, the study of wildlife, art, amateur dramatics or in cultural or religious activities enables children effortlessly to learn from them. They acquire their parents' knowledge and skills in the opportunities that arise naturally and if they can belong to a wider network of people all with a common interest in and commitment to that activity, so the range of models for young people to emulate is broadened.

Emotional and sexual development, occurring during these years, do make conflict between parents and offspring more likely, but expressing confidence in young people and arriving at shared decisions about, for example, coming-in times, clothes, chores in the household, time spent texting and phoning friends can all increase good communication and mutual respect. Appendix 12 provides a template for an agreement which can be arrived at either within the family unit or with the assistance of a helping person.

CLOSE SUPERVISION OF THE YOUNG PERSON'S WHEREABOUTS

The studies of Wilson and of Farrington, mentioned above, highlight the crucial importance of parents spending time with and supervising their young people, *starting not now in the early teenage years, but from toddlerhood and throughout childhood.* Many, many studies have investigated the relationship between parenting and subsequent delinquency, and in their meta-analysis Hoeve *et al.* (2009) quote this conclusion: 'Among the over seventy studies reviewed, the best predictors of delinquency and problem behavior included lack of parental supervision, parent rejection and [low] parent–child involvement… (Loeber and Stouthamer-Loeber 1986)'.

Since, however, we wish to focus on protective factors, we will reiterate that parents will be wise to keep in close touch with their young people, to build relationships with their children's friends, to invite them for meals or outings, to make it clear what time they are expected to be home, to sanction them if they do not come at the specified time, to refuse to go out when young people want to bring their friends home for an evening party even though the young people make a great fuss, to provide an example of how much alcohol, if any, to drink, and to follow through on any privileges and/or sanctions which have been made clear beforehand. It does children no favours to give them unlimited freedom in their teenage years.

Reducing risks of gang involvement

Every city is likely to have large numbers of gangs of young people who come together for a sense of belonging, excitement and easy rewards. Older gang members are likely to be on the lookout for recruits, often youngsters in their early teens, who can act as junior members and who can swell the numbers of the gang and thus its earning capacity. So what can parents and teachers do to prevent children from joining gangs? [9] As we have discussed above, children who have good relationships with their parents and wider families from their earliest years are likely to be among those who take advantage of opportunities at school, develop warm friendships and make contributions to their communities. They are less likely to find gang membership attractive. Box 5.1 shows some specific suggestions for what parents can do to help.

---

9   See www.helpingamericasyouth.gov

Box 5.1 Suggestions for parents on discouraging gang membership

- Talk to and listen to your child from early childhood onwards. Spend some special time with each child.
- Discourage harassing/bullying behaviours.
- Put a high value on education and help your child to do his or her best in school. Do everything possible to prevent dropping out. Talk to staff at school frequently about your child's progress and how you can support this.
- Do not criticise the young person's teachers or school in his hearing. If you have concerns, go to the teacher or the school head.
- Help your child identify positive role models and heroes – especially people in your community. If you are active in the community and people look up to you, your child is likely to wish to be like you.
- Do everything possible to involve your child in supervised, positive group activities.
- Praise them for doing well and encourage them to do their very best – to stretch their skills to the uttermost.
- Know what your children are doing and with whom. Know about their friends and their friends' families.
- Talk to your child and discuss the consequences of being a gang member.
- Seek advice from religious leaders or community mentors.
- Report and remove graffiti from your neighbourhood.
- Take action, listen to and communicate with your child.

PARENTING/CHILD MANAGEMENT SKILLS TRAINING

Although it is simpler and less demanding to work with the parents of young children in helping them with their child management skills, the evidence is that good success can be achieved with the parents of older children. Both *The Incredible Years* (Webster-Stratton 1992) and the *Triple P* (Sanders 1999) approaches have developed versions of their programmes targeted at children of up to age 14: the former has developed a package entitled 'Dinosaur' which focuses on children aged 7–11 who exhibit ongoing conduct problems and/or symptoms of ADHD, while versions of the *Triple P* package have also demonstrated efficacy for this age range. Functional Family Therapy (FFT) is a programme for which there is considerable evidence of success with young people aged 11 onwards. Lane *et al.* (2004) summarise the approach of FFT as shown in Box 5.2.

Box 5.2 Treatment phases in Functional Family Therapy

Risk factors are targeted in three treatment phases that build towards a process of positive change:

- Phase 1 focuses on reducing negative communication and hopelessness and increasing the motivation of family members to participate in change.

- Phase 2 focuses on developing and implementing individualised behaviour change plans.

- Phase 3 focuses on helping families to generalise positive changes to other problems or situations they encounter.

Several studies using the FFT approach have demonstrated marked improvements in family interactions and reduced levels of offending by both the young people and their younger siblings (Alexander and Parsons 1980; Ghate and Ramella 2002).

These and other parenting packages have all successfully demonstrated that with ongoing support and training in child management skills, it is possible for skilled and committed workers to help parents to learn to achieve major improvements in family life for themselves and their children in this age group. The results of a meta-analysis of eight smaller evaluations of FFT undertaken by Aos *et al.* (2011) showed that this is a cost-effective approach for reducing juvenile crime. Moreover, longitudinal studies, which have followed up the families in general and the young people in particular, have shown that these improvements can maintain for as long as five years after the end of active support. Programmes of FFT are now being disseminated in the UK.

All the programmes, by teaching tried and tested ways of interacting among family members, such as identifying positive features of behaviour and highlighting strengths rather than weaknesses, help participants learn and rehearse appreciative interactions rather than hostile and critical ones. These programmes all make use of well-established principles of social learning theory, explored in earlier chapters.

DEVISING WRITTEN AGREEMENTS

There is a great deal of evidence that a key skill of practitioners seeking to help families in difficulties is writing individualised agreements with the young person concerned and with family members. This may seem an unusual activity for many parents who are more familiar with patterns of parenting where Dad or Mum says what is to happen and the child or young person has to comply – or there is major trouble. However, the evidence is that a great deal can be achieved if, as children mature, they are brought to participate in discussion about difficulties and in agreeing how they may be resolved. Box 5.3 shows essential steps in devising an agreement.

A template for such an agreement is included as Appendix 12.

Box 5.3 Essential steps in devising an agreement (after Sheldon 1980)

1.   Discuss whether an agreement is socially acceptable to those involved. It may be familiar for business arrangements, but not for personal ones. If so, invite people to try the idea out.

2.   Focus on actions or behaviours rather than on attitudes or feelings. Select one or two behaviours initially. Avoid working with too many problems. Early success is vital.

---

3. Describe those behaviours in a very clear way. The behaviour should be observable by anyone watching and people should be able to agree on the basis of what they have observed that it did or did not happen. For example:

    - a child did or did not attend school
    - a parent did or did not invite a young person's friends for a meal
    - the young person did or did not help clear up after a meal.

4. Write the agreement so that everyone understands it. Make the wording clear, brief and simple and written in each person's first language. Information can be recorded daily on simple charts such as lists and rotas.

5. Everyone must gain something from the agreement. The benefits for each person must be worth the costs. An agreement is *not* a list of rules.

6. The language should be positive – specifying behaviours which are to be carried out, rather than behaviours which must not be carried out. For example, 'Everyone to speak as they'd like to be spoken to', rather than 'No swearing'.

7. Collect records. It is essential to know whether the situation is getting better or not.

8. Renegotiate the agreement after, say, one week. A series of short-term agreements is generally more effective than one long-term one.

9. If there is going to be a penalty for failure to fulfil an agreement, this must be made clear at the outset: for example, if pocket money is going to be withheld if certain behaviours are not carried out.

10. Everyone concerned must sign the agreement. Try to involve all concerned when devising it.

A STRONG SCHOOL ETHOS: BACKING SCHOOL STANDARDS

There has been substantial research to identify the characteristics of effective schools. The seminal text *Fifteen Thousand Hours* (Rutter *et al.* 1979) explored the impact on children of features of their secondary school experience, and identified eight main characteristics of effective schools (Box 5.4).

Box 5.4 Main characteristics of effective schools (Rutter *et al.* 1979)

- A strong, positive school ethos (the characteristic spirit of a school as shown in its attitudes and aspirations)
- Effective classroom management
- High teacher expectations
- Teachers as positive role models
- Positive feedback and treatment of students
- Good working conditions for staff and students
- Students given responsibility
- Shared staff–student activities.

While other researchers have identified additional or slightly different variables, the above list has frequently been confirmed in subsequent studies. Other researchers are increasingly citing good relationships between school staff and parents as a valuable feature of effective schools, and although in the UK there are few staff employed exclusively to liaise with parents, school nurses can and do fulfil an invaluable role in linking home and school.

There is further encouraging evidence that schools can contribute substantially to enhancing the wellbeing of young people. Perra *et al.* (2012, p.1), associated with the Belfast Youth Development Study, report:

The two factors which were consistently and independently associated with regular substance use among both males and females were student–teacher relationships and fighting at school: positive teacher relationships reduced the risk of daily smoking by 48%, weekly drunkenness by 25% and weekly cannabis use by 52%; being in a fight increased the risk of daily smoking by 54%, weekly drunkenness by 31% and weekly cannabis use by 43%.

With such impressively high levels of reductions of use of dangerous substances by young people in their early teens, associated with positive relationships with teachers, further research must surely be focused on promoting such relationships among students and their teachers in secondary schools.

MENTORING PROGRAMMES

Since truancy seems to be a frequent precursor of substance abuse, it is extremely important to try to retain young people in school. Many schools make Herculean efforts to work with the young people themselves, as well as with their parents, through school nurses, counsellors and youth workers but resources for such work are increasingly limited. One approach which has had a measure of success in the UK has been mentoring, and a recent advisory document by O'Connor and Waddell (2015) gives information and advice to those commissioning mentoring programmes. They offer the following: 'Often, mentoring is defined as a one-to-one, non-judgemental relationship in which an individual (the "mentor") gives time to support and encourage another (the "mentee"). Mentors may offer direct assistance, such as help with job searching, and/or indirect support through encouragement, acting as a positive role model, and challenging the mentee's views, for example.'

These researchers refer to two specific evaluations of mentoring. The first, a review and meta-analysis by Tolan *et al.* (2008), found that, overall, high-risk young people, already at risk of future delinquency, who were allocated mentors displayed a lower likelihood of delinquency, aggression and drug use and achieved better academic outcomes than those who were not mentored. Effects were stronger when emotional support was a key part of the mentoring provision. The second, by Jolliffe and Farrington (2007), found that mentoring had a significant beneficial influence in reducing subsequent offending for young people at risk of offending or who had been involved with the police compared with those without mentors. Overall there was a 10 per cent reduction in offending by those young people who had mentors. The best results were where mentor and mentee spent more time together and where other interventions were available to the young person as well. However, the benefits of mentoring did not always continue after the mentoring ended.

These reviews indicate that careful thought and planning needs to be given to the content of mentoring activities, the mentors' motivation for involvement and the frequency and duration of meetings. Those planning to develop a mentoring service should study the recommendations provided by O'Connor and Waddell, as well as the useful checklists provided.

In the United States, the organisation Big Brothers, Big Sisters (BBBS) is 'committed to improving the life-chances of at-risk children and teens' by providing each young person with an adult friend. The mentors met with the young people three or four times a month on average for about three hours a time for at least a year. An evaluation carried out by Grossman and Tierney (1998) at eight sites across the USA and involving more than 1100 young people participating in the programme as well as a control group who had no mentors found that the young people with mentors were significantly less likely to have hit someone (32% less), embarked on illegal drug use (46% less), become involved in alcohol use (27% less) or truanted from school (30% less). Aos et al. (2011) found that for every dollar spent on the programme more than three dollars were saved to the government and crime victims. A BBBS programme has now been set up in London.

There is encouraging news also from Australia concerning the use of the internet to reduce truancy and associated psychological distress. A randomised controlled trial was carried out by Newton et al. (2009) in Australia to assess the outcomes of a course aimed at reducing alcohol and cannabis use with a package comprising two sets of six lessons given about six months apart. Some 764 students with a mean age of 13.1 years from ten schools were randomly allocated to a preventive intervention or their usual classes on maintaining good health. Measures were taken at pre-intervention, post-intervention and some six and twelve months following the intervention. Not only did the strategy help reduce alcohol and cannabis use, but students in the intervention group showed reduced truancy and psychological distress up to twelve months following the end of the intervention. Such internet-based strategies are likely to become far more popular.

MULTISYSTEMIC THERAPY

These programmes focus on multiple factors or systems contributing to antisocial behaviour. In the United States many have been shown by rigorous evaluation to be successful. The aims of the practitioners are:

- to help young people break links with violent peers
- to help young people build strong links with family and school members
- to enhance parents' family management skills such as monitoring young people's behaviour
- to develop the young person's academic and social competencies.

The approach clearly has much in common with FFT. Each young person and his or her family members are engaged in an individualised plan, and the wellbeing of the parents as well as the young person is addressed. Members of the social networks of the family are engaged to support the participants. The key components and strategies of the programme are taught to the family members over five days and 'booster sessions' are offered every three months. Further information can be found at the programme's website.[10]

Specialist training for the practitioners is necessary, but with trained workers great improvements, including reduced offending and lower levels of mental health problems, have been found for the young people while family functioning has also improved. The approach is being exhaustively trialled in the UK.

---

10 www.mstuk.org

Theoretical underpinnings of multisystemic therapy

As the title of the approach implies, practitioners are trained in systems thinking and envisage the young person and his or her parents and siblings as involved in many different social and other networks: family, community, economic and social. They work with family members as participants in their efforts to help all concerned, and it is these family members who set the treatment goals with the young person and for themselves. Multisystemic therapists are guided by the principles listed in Box 5.5 (Henggeler *et al.* 1998).

Box 5.5 Principles underpinning multisystemic therapy

1. *Finding the fit.* The primary purpose of assessment is to understand how the influences from various systems contribute to and make sense of the difficulties experienced by the young person. For example, how resistance to pressure from school to attend each morning at 9.00a.m. may lead to a young person being seen as rebellious, which in turn leads him to associate with other young people who are alienated from school.

2. *Positive and strengths focused.* Therapeutic contacts emphasise the positive and use participants' strengths as levers for change.

3. *Increasing responsibility.* Interventions are designed to promote responsible behaviour among family members.

4. *Present-focused, action-oriented and well-defined.* Interventions focus on current situations, are action-oriented, target-specific and they define problems tightly.

5. *Targeting sequences.* Interventions target sequences of behaviour within or between multiple systems that maintain the identified problems, for example the link between a morning argument between father and son and the young person not reaching school on time.

6. *Developmentally appropriate.* Interventions fit the developmental needs of the young people.

7. *Continuous effort.* Interventions are designed to require daily or weekly effort by family members.

---

8. *Evaluation and accountability.* Intervention effectiveness is evaluated continuously from multiple perspectives, with providers assuming accountability for overcoming barriers to successful outcomes.

9. *Generalisation.* Interventions are designed to promote treatment generalisation and long-term maintenance of therapeutic change by empowering caregivers to address family members' needs across many systems.

USING COGNITIVE BEHAVIOURAL PRINCIPLES IN WORK WITH PARENTS

The term cognitive behavioural therapy (CBT) is becoming part of everyday language, and we explored core beliefs and Negative Automatic Thoughts briefly in Chapter 2. The name refers to a way in which professionally trained practitioners can help people to distinguish their beliefs about themselves and the world and whether these are accurate and helpful to them. Abundant research, developing the work of Aaron Beck, the founder of formal cognitive psychology, has shown that enabling people to reflect on their core beliefs has freed them to become aware of those beliefs and, as appropriate, to question them. For example, here are a number of deeply held beliefs of parents with whom I have worked:

- I grew up in care, so I shall never be able to look after a child.
- I must never let my child's bid for attention be ignored. I must always attend to him.
- It would be rude not to answer Sebastian's question, however often he asks.
- Children who are praised will get a big head.
- If I'm in prison, it must be because of bad blood.

These beliefs emerged in the course of our discussions about a child's wild and disruptive behaviour or about themselves: I did not deliberately ask about them. If this situation arises, that is, if a deep different belief is stated in response to, say, our suggestion that a child benefits from hearing regular positive feedback for trying hard, or that a rude and unpleasant comment by a child should just be ignored, one can ask gently where the parent learned that particular principle or whether there might be any exceptions to the rule. Our queries need, of course, to be informed by our own understanding of theory and should be suggestions, even musings, not outright challenges. The point is that unless we have had specific training in principles of cognitive behavioural theory, we should confine ourselves to gentle queries rather than getting into deep water by actively challenging parents' views.

OTHER APPROACHES WITH A STRONG EVIDENCE BASE
A problem-solving approach

This approach lends itself to the resolution of many difficulties, concerning older children and teenagers as well as adults. In essence, the process requires that a difficulty should be fully explored and then formulated as a 'problem-to-be-solved'. The process was originally expressed as in Box 5.6.

Box 5.6 Steps of the problem-solving process (Spivack, Platt and Shure 1976)

1. Pinpoint the problem.

2. Gather as much information about the problem as possible.

3. Express the difficulty in terms of a problem-to-be-solved.

4. Generate potential solutions by means of a 'brainstorm'. Any ideas, however fanciful, may be put forward; criticism is deliberately withheld.

5. Examine the potential outcomes of each solution. How well does each one solve the problem? What would be happening if a solution could be found?

6. Agree on the best strategy/solution.

7. Plan how to implement the strategy.

---

8. Put the plan into action.

9. Review and evaluate the effectiveness of the plan. If unsuccessful, adapt it or try another strategy from the list generated earlier. Repeat these steps until a solution is found.

An example of problem solving

Gary has a diagnosis of ADHD. It can be managed if Gary takes his medication, usually Ritalin, regularly. His mother gives him a dose before he leaves home for school in the mornings, but he needs to take another dose in school – and it is this that he usually 'forgets'. Different solutions to this difficulty are explored and it is agreed that his mother will approach his class teacher to see if an arrangement can be made whereby the school nurse or a designated teacher gives Gary his medication at an agreed time – so allowing Gary to concentrate calmly in the classroom instead of being constantly active and disruptive.

The potential of Teen Online Problem Solving (TOPS) approaches

The potential of the internet for contributing to the management or resolution of human difficulties is only just beginning to be explored. Among the initiatives which are being developed and rigorously evaluated are programmes to address parent–teenager conflict. The TOPS package has been developed to help counter the difficulties which arise among teenagers who have sustained traumatic brain injury (TBI).

Several studies have investigated the impact of this online initiative on the improvement of the injured young peoples' executive function – a term which refers to our cognitive abilities to hold information in mind, to plan, organise and regulate our activities. These abilities are of course central to basic life skills and if the brain processes underpinning them are prejudiced by brain damage then the young person's skills in problem solving, communication and self-regulation are likely to be greatly reduced. Brain injuries are also likely to contribute to conflict between the young person and his or her caregivers.

The specially designed training programmes administered online have brought very encouraging outcomes for the young people and their caregivers. Wade *et al.* (2011), who worked with 41 young people who had all experienced TBI, found that those in the group who received the TOPS training demonstrated marked improvements by comparison with those who experienced a less focused training using the general resources of the internet. The researchers report that when differing backgrounds and degrees of brain injury among the young people had been controlled for, 'the TOPS group reported significantly less parent–teen conflict at follow-up than did the internet-resource comparison group.' While brain-injured young people are a small, specialist group, the success which they experienced using the online programme suggests that it will not be long before similar packages are developed to assist with reducing conflict among teenagers and their parents in the general population.

CHAPTER 6

Summary and Cross-Cutting Themes

OVERVIEW

- Cumulative risk: the impact of poverty and disadvantage
- The protective contribution of relationships: parents' bonding with their baby
- The protective contribution of relationships: baby's attachment to parents
- The impact of parenting styles: principles from social learning theory
- Talking and reading to babies, toddlers and children
- The importance of fathers and grandparents: involvement in children's activities
- Close supervision of children's activities: start young!
- Encouraging self-control by the child
- Facilitating close relationships with nurseries, playgroups and schools
- The helping person as positive model, coach and architect of success

After all the confusion and uncertainty which in previous centuries has characterised research into children's difficulties, such as poor mental health, failure to achieve potential at school and becoming involved in patterns of offending, we are now at last in the twenty-first century beginning to gain some real understanding of the risk and protective factors which impinge on children and young people, of the way in which risk accumulates and how children and families can surmount risks and enhance wellbeing. The evidence is getting better and better: studies from around the world are converging on key sets of circumstances and conditions which pose threats and others which offer support. This final chapter will summarise these cross-cutting themes. However, we have explained throughout that our intention is, while acknowledging risk factors, to focus primarily on protective factors and on what people who wish to give help and support to families with young children can offer to achieve this.

CUMULATIVE RISK: THE IMPACT OF POVERTY AND DISADVANTAGE

Children born into poor homes are likely to encounter markedly greater challenges than children from more advantaged backgrounds and these difficulties deepen as they get older. Abundant studies across the Western world have demonstrated that neglected neighbourhoods, impoverished backgrounds and limited social cohesion all contribute to children starting education at a marked disadvantage and that the differences between them and more advantaged children widen as they get older. In these impoverished settings children are unable to flourish or to achieve their potential. It is not only the absence of facilities and resources which is damaging, but also the stress caused by lack of money, isolation, and lack of support which sap parents' abilities to provide loving and stable homes for their children.

Some children do come into the world with characteristics which make it more likely that they will have difficulties: for example, some seem to be at a genetic risk of ADHD and this, interacting with environmental factors, appears to strengthen the probability that they will encounter problems and, in the most challenging scenarios, they may become involved in offending. For we have seen that *risk accumulates*: young people do not suddenly without any warning signs embark overnight on a criminal career; on the contrary, there are plenty of earlier signs which should raise our concern. Often we *do* experience concern, but there are not the resources to respond to them.

We see from Figure I.1 the variables which at each developmental stage are hazardous for the child or young person, and a model of cumulative risk serves best to capture the number and range of those hazards. It follows, therefore, that if risk accumulates then the removal or reduction of even one of those risks, or the provision of some small element of protection, may be enough to give that child a better life trajectory and to enhance his or her wellbeing.

THE PROTECTIVE CONTRIBUTION OF RELATIONSHIPS: PARENTS' BONDING WITH THEIR BABY

We have seen that during early pregnancy initial levels of oxytocin, usually associated with bonding and caregiving, predicted mothers' levels of bonding behaviour with their infants: this was measured by touching, gazing at and gentle talk to the infant. So mothers are partially prepared by Nature for their maternal role and should not be blamed if they do not immediately 'fall in love' with their babies. However, with support from nursing and other caregivers and, it is to be hoped, during the course of breastfeeding, the emotions associated with bonding with the baby intensify, underpinned by hormonal processes, and the protective and loving impulses that are intended by Nature blossom and flourish. This process, including breastfeeding, can of course be supported or undermined by the father. We saw that domestic violence or abuse is particularly damaging not just to the mother but also prejudices her relationship with her baby; but if the father cares for the child, smiling at her, bathing her and playing with her, then he is likely to feel the same bonding emotions as the mother. In particular, if he encourages breastfeeding, then the way is clearer for this highly desirable activity to become established and he is doing a great service both to his child and to his partner.

We have seen from the research of Odgers *et al.* (2012) that supportive parenting, that is, warmth, affection, praise and clear guidance, can offset the impact of widening socioeconomic disparities during middle childhood. The study focused on children of ages five to 12, the very period when children are beginning to encounter the wider world of school and its associated challenges. This is a particularly valuable study, in that it indicates that the protective impact of confident and authoritative parenting can exert its influence far beyond the particular period commonly regarded as supremely important, namely the first five years. If practitioners can recognise the need for support of parents in these primary school years as well as in early childhood, can build on their strengths, enhance their bonding with the child, and if necessary offer them skills of nurturing and managing their children, then many of the risks posed by difficulties in the early years can be offset.

THE PROTECTIVE CONTRIBUTION OF RELATIONSHIPS: BABY'S ATTACHMENT TO PARENTS

Nature has so arranged infant development that it is not normally until about the middle of the first year of life that babies begin to distinguish their main caregiver, often but not always the mother, as the person with whom they feel safe and with whom they wish to spend most of their time. They have, as we say, become attached. There may be several people with whom the baby develops attachments – indeed, it is desirable that there should be, in case the mother or main caregiver falls sick or for whatever reason cannot care for the child – so, following Fahlberg (1988), we speak of a hierarchy of attachments, often with the mother at the top. These primary relationships are profoundly significant: they enable the baby to survive emotionally in a dangerous world and to feel the security of that person's protectiveness throughout infancy, childhood and into adolescence and adulthood.

However, levels of attachment are not fixed once and for all in infancy or early childhood: an attachment which began as insecure can become secure as the child experiences love and affection either from his own parents if they can be helped to respond to his needs, or from foster or adoptive parents if care by his natural parents is not possible. We can see the types of experiences which can contribute to that increasing security in Appendix 4 (Silverstein 1996). What isn't known is how many changes of foster or adoptive parents can be made before the child's capacity to make trusting relationships is damaged irreparably. When we read of children who have had many, many moves within the childcare system, we must wonder about their resilience. Of course, many children for whom adoptive parents are sought have complex needs: they have physical or emotional disabilities, they have features of ADHD or they have experienced trauma in this country or overseas. Yet even for these, it is remarkable what healing the regular provision of ongoing love and care can achieve in helping a child gain security and confidence to cope with the demands of school and day-to day living.

THE IMPACT OF PARENTING STYLES: PRINCIPLES FROM SOCIAL LEARNING THEORY

We have seen that certain styles of parenting, notably a harsh and rejecting pattern of interaction with the child, are particularly damaging to him or her and may be reflected in serious misbehaviour both at home and at school. And we have seen that neglect, which may stem from parental depression or substance misuse, also actively harms the child. By contrast, an authoritative and warm style of parenting, with clear guidance given to the child about how he or she should behave, with boundaries firmly in place and approval when he complies is known to lead to confidence in the child and a clear sense of security. 'I'm not allowed' can be a very helpful message for parents to teach their children to announce when some bad behaviour or diversion is suggested in the primary school playground.

To reiterate the research conclusion in this area: whatever the challenges faced by children, whether they grow up in difficult and disadvantaged circumstances or in more affluent ones, the impact of warm and supportive parenting is paramount. As Odgers and her colleagues (2012) explain, by the term 'supportive parenting' is meant 'maternal warmth and parental monitoring' of behaviour and activities.

When helping parents to develop firm but loving ways of interacting with their children, social learning theory offers some invaluable principles. These are well-tried and underpin many of the parenting packages which are now available. A small team of us at De Montfort University are teaching a principle derived from social learning theory, namely, giving frequent and regular praise. The 'Give a Child 5 Praises a Day' campaign and a card illustrating this approach is shown in Appendix 7. We ask parents to 'Catch them being good' and to give positive reinforcement or feedback to the child on at least five occasions each day. Preliminary results, both quantitative and qualitative, are very encouraging.

TALKING AND READING TO BABIES, TODDLERS AND CHILDREN

During the early years parents can give enormous impetus to the child's cognitive development particularly simply by talking to him or her: chatting as they go out and about or round the house, pointing out colours and shapes; exploring things in the natural world such as leaves, flowers, insects and minibeasts. This is the age in which wonder can be conveyed, together with the language to accompany the miracle of rainbows, the sloppiness of jelly and the messiness of mud. This is the period too when parents and children can delight in singing, nursery rhymes and tongue twisters and when music and dance can convey balance, rhythm and imaginative movement. Children of every age seem to love riddles, jingles, and poems with silly words and meanings. I remember my own delight in the poem *Jabberwocky* when introduced to it in primary school and how it revealed to me that words were not fixed and final, but could be made up. This pleasure has lasted all my life.

With the tensions between loyalties to home and to peer groups gaining strength during this time, school work may suffer, so it is extremely encouraging to read the most recent data concerning primary school children undergoing the Standard Attainment Tests (SATs) in England. These show that there has been an improvement of four percentage points in the proportion of children aged 11 who achieved a level 4 or above in reading, writing and mathematics: in 2013 only 75 per cent of children reached this level; in 2014, 79 per cent of children did so (Department for Education 2014b). This improvement reflects huge commitment and investment of time and encouragement by thousands of teachers, language specialists, play workers, teachers, classroom assistants and parents and is a wonderful achievement!

THE IMPORTANCE OF FATHERS AND GRANDPARENTS: INVOLVEMENT IN CHILDREN'S ACTIVITIES

We saw when exploring how a home visitor may be able to support parents-to-be during pregnancy that while the mother will probably be the focus of our main attention we should be careful to include the father and, where appropriate, the grandparents in our efforts to be supportive to the family. The evidence is clear that many fathers do wish to be part of discussions and planning, but are all too often left on the sidelines. However, it is evident that researchers have neglected fathers and their contributions to the wellbeing of their children, though the work of Ramchandani and his team (2013) is demonstrating that the significance of fathers for their children's wellbeing is often as great as that of mothers. It seems it may be particularly important for boys.

A related field is the advantages which can accrue to children if parents and grandparents can be involved in their activities and if, as families, they have some shared interests: sport, camping, fishing, art, music, drama or the hundred and one other pastimes which are usually available to many families. While children may complain about being expected to accompany other family members to dog training sessions or to camping expeditions, when what they really want to do is to watch television, it seems that to have a field of interest in which many family members are routinely involved from early childhood can be extremely valuable. This not only provides everyone with knowledge and experience which they can share with other members of the extended family, but also it gives children a ready-made network of friends all interested in wildlife or climbing Munros. I remember that our third child, not particularly interested at the age of ten in outdoor pursuits, when asked what he would like for a Christmas present, groaned, 'I suppose I'd better ask for a tent!' He did, the tent arrived, and he slept in it for countless camps and expeditions. In due course he became a hill-walker and climber himself.

CLOSE SUPERVISION OF CHILDREN'S ACTIVITIES: START YOUNG!

Throughout their development parents should monitor *very closely* the whereabouts of their young children. Rules about going out and coming back, who they are with and where the child is at any time in the day should be made and practised by all concerned during these primary school years. The parents can provide an example by setting out their own plans for the day and how these may affect the children. This not only models responsible behaviour by the parents but also sets up habits of communication which can be invaluable later. Waiting until the child is moving into secondary school is far too late.

In Chapter 5, concerning children of nine to thirteen, we saw that authoritative parenting, where firm control is exercised over children's activities when out of the house, is central for their wellbeing. They can of course enjoy as much freedom as the parents feel is safe, but it is the supervision and the knowledge of where they are, who they are with and when they will be back which is so crucial. For, as we saw, it is during this period that children's loyalties may shift from the parents towards peers and school friends and with this shift may go a shift of tastes, attitudes and habits.

ENCOURAGING SELF-CONTROL BY THE CHILD

We saw in Chapter 4 the evidence that encouraging the child to take responsibility for decisions that are within his capability, and for parents, where possible, to support those decisions, is likely to lead to children becoming self-motivating and self-reliant. So, for example, we saw that giving pocket money, and making it clear what has to come out of this sum, can lead to children learning early in life how quickly money disappears and that to save up for expensive items is a valuable habit.

Within our own family, following advice from parents with older children, we managed most weeks to have a weekly family meeting, lasting about 20 minutes. Matters which affected everybody, like who would care for our hamster when we went on holiday and whether a friend could come for a sleepover, were discussed, and the children, then aged about five and seven, gave their views loudly. There was also a toddler, but we didn't get his view! I remember one particular occasion when my husband and I were wondering whether to become foster parents to a three-year-old. We were surprised how maturely our two children thought about the idea, and while we, as parents, carried the full responsibility for the decision, it was good to realise that children still in primary school were in agreement. The outcome was that we went ahead and were foster parents for two years before adopting our foster child.

FACILITATING CLOSE RELATIONSHIPS WITH NURSERIES, PLAYGROUPS AND SCHOOLS

Close liaison between home and nursery or home and school is invaluable. Huge resources have been ploughed into providing wonderful activities for young children, as well as many involving parents, for several hours a week in nurseries or Children's Centres. Now many centres will also offer places for two-year-olds. Although the cost of childcare is threatening the ability of many families to pay for it, the opportunities offered to young children in other settings are still rich and life-enhancing. For if children move easily into playgroups and settle well there, these experiences provide them with the confidence and achievements to enhance their subsequent life chances. As we have seen, there is evidence that this early investment is beginning to bring results.

We also saw that this is the age during which language and literacy can be painlessly promoted and encouraged. Taking children to libraries so that they can see adults engrossed in books, or attending story-telling sessions in Children's Centres, are enriching experiences, as is inventing stories about people whom the parent and child see when they are out together: where that man comes from; what that woman's name might be; why she is wearing a green hat; whether he has any children; whether she will catch the bus she is running for; who takes the dog for a walk; whether it will rain later in the day. All these themes can be explored while on the bus or while walking back from the shops.

THE HELPING PERSON AS POSITIVE MODEL, COACH AND ARCHITECT OF SUCCESS

So much rests on relationships. As we have insisted throughout this book, we shall not be allowed across the threshold unless we can convey to the families we are trying to help our empathy, our genuineness, our respect for them and our feelings of warmth towards them. These are fundamental principles in our approach to all those concerned: parents, grandparents, children and all family members. If our approach is guided by these principles, sincerely held, then we may be able to avoid triggering the threat-detection systems centring on the amygdala within the brain's limbic system.

A second principle for practice which cuts across many settings in which we as helpers may find ourselves is that of attending to the strengths and potentials of those we encounter. As reported, practitioners of solution-focused approaches actively teach their students to start their meetings with clients by giving a compliment – but to those who find this too contrived and 'false', we can respond, as we saw above, that there is substantial evidence that incorporating a 'strengths-based' element in counselling or psychotherapy has been shown to lead to beneficial outcomes. This is perhaps an echo of the maxim 'accentuate the positive' so often cited in management manuals.

So, while visiting a family which spends much of the available time complaining about either their personal circumstances or about their offspring, it may well be appropriate, after allowing the complaints to run their necessary stress-relieving course – I think my longest 'just listening' interval lasted an hour – to ask what positive features of their situation or the behaviour of the same child the family can identify. We may have to work to extract this information from them, but it does provide a fallback scenario which we, in need of finding something, *anything*, positive in an otherwise apparently hopeless situation, can serve to revive the spirits of all concerned. When I am feeling depressed about the small number of families where I have been able to achieve a real improvement in family life and in relieving the depression of the parents, I still return to a handful of settings where I know, and have evidence, that circumstances are markedly improved. As mentioned earlier, I even have a few letters, now tattered, that I read and re-read to lift my spirits in discouraging times.

Overall, then, there is a heartening convergence of evidence for the value of 'accentuating the positive', of enabling the home visitor to act as support person and architect of success for those whom he or she visits. Such people of course, as we have insisted, if they are not themselves senior and professionally qualified, will need regular and skilled supervision so that they identify situations where referrals to other services beyond their own are necessary. But working by 'baby steps' towards achievable goals is a wonderful way of working. If these principles are observed, and if the armies of volunteers which Britain offers continue to come forward, then with even modest resources the wellbeing of children and their parents can continue to be enhanced.

Maternal Confidence Questionnaire (Dilmore 2004)

This questionnaire should be used for discussion, rather than as a scored instrument. It could be used on several occasions, e.g. one month, three months and six months after the birth of the baby.

**How confident do you feel in your parenting role?
(Mark appropriate box)**

		Never	Seldom	Sometimes	Often	A great deal
1	I know when my baby wants me to play with him/her					
2	I know how to take care of my baby better than anyone else					

	Never	Seldom	Sometimes	Often	A great deal
3	When my baby is cranky, I know the reason				
4	I can tell when my baby is tired and needs to sleep				
5	I know what makes my baby happy				
6	I can give my baby a bath				
7	I can feed my baby adequately				
8	I can hold my baby properly				
9	I can tell when my baby is sick				

10	I feel frustrated taking care of my baby				
11	I would be good at helping other mothers learn how to take care of their infants				
12	Being a parent is demanding and unrewarding				
13	I have all the skills needed to be a good parent				
14	I am satisfied with my role as a parent				

A simple scale to indicate bonding (after Silverstein 1996)

Such a scale could be used for both mothers and fathers to indicate their current feeling of bonding with their baby – say monthly.

1. I don't feel close at all
2. I don't feel close
3. I feel medium
4. I feel a little bit close
5. I feel close
6. I feel really close

The Postpartum Bonding Instrument (Brockington 2001)

Again, this should be used for discussion, rather than as a scored instrument, and can be completed every few months.

Please tick the appropriate box

		Always	Very often	Quite often	Sometimes	Rarely	Never
1	I feel close to my baby						
2	I wish the old days when I had no baby would come back						
3	I feel distant from my baby						
4	I love to cuddle my baby						
5	I regret having this baby						

		Always	Very often	Quite often	Sometimes	Rarely	Never
6	The baby does not seem to be mine						
7	My baby winds me up						
8	My baby irritates me						
9	I feel happy when my baby smiles or laughs						
10	I love my baby to bits						
11	I enjoy playing with my baby						
12	My baby cries too much						
13	I feel trapped as a mother						
14	I feel angry with my baby						
15	I resent my baby						
16	My baby is the most beautiful baby in the world						

17	I wish my baby would somehow go away				
18	I have done harmful things to my baby				
19	My baby makes me anxious				
20	I am afraid of my baby				
21	My baby annoys me				
22	I feel confident when changing my baby				
23	I feel the only solution is for someone else to look after my baby				
24	I feel like hurting my baby				
25	My baby is easily comforted				

Ways of increasing family attachment (after Silverstein 1996)

PRINCIPLES GUIDING THE PROCESSES OF INCREASING FAMILY ATTACHMENT

They are experiential, but theory based

They enhance the ability of parents or carers to offer the child comfort, safety and security: the aim is to reduce anxiety

They are usually based in some form of play

They allow the child to regress and feel/behave as a younger child

They increase parents' own confidence, and enjoyment of the child

1 Holding/touch

Rocking and holding, with gentle touching, singing, stroking

Bottle-feeding for a few minutes each day for young children

Counting fingers and toes

Massaging, applying lotion

Lap time – have child on lap for a few minutes night and morning

2 Play

Doll play: feeding, cuddling, dressing and undressing, bathing

Balls and balloons: rolling to and fro

Taking turns in games

Hide and seek: peekaboo

Making faces: copying sad and happy faces, surprise, delight

Singing nursery rhymes, songs

Art: scribbling, crayons, paints

3 Feelings education

Making faces, sounds about feelings: cross, unhappy,

Talk about feelings of others in story books or on TV

Show how natural feelings are: fear, joy, anger

Bring dollies close and then take them apart: how do they feel?

4 Heightening opportunities to nurture

Activities involving soothing, calming, reassuring

Child sits by parent(s) at meal times: touch and talk to child

Nurse child when sick; empathise with feelings – you're not feeling well

Give special time and attention

Allow child to cry and accept comfort

Bedtime routines to strengthen security

5 Clarification of life events (if appropriate)

Child needs to understand, in a simple way, what has happened to them and that they are blameless

Life-story books, with photographs of key people in previous settings

Visits to people and places formerly familiar to them, with simple explanations according to age

Future planning so that the child knows what is likely to happen in the future: for example, is this a 'forever family' or not?

6 Activities which highlight identification with family (if appropriate)

Involving child in family traditions: birthdays, bedtime, visits, holidays

Involving relatives in caring for child

7 Discipline

Set firm, consistent boundaries

Avoid strategies which involve separation or loss

Use techniques which can be shared with another family member: for example, washing up

Make punishments brief and relevant: get them over and done with

Activities to encourage speech and language development

(With acknowledgements to the American Speech, Language and Hearing Association.)

BIRTH TO 2 YEARS

- Encourage your baby to make vowel-like and consonant–vowel sounds such as 'ma', 'da', and 'ba'.

- Reinforce attempts by maintaining eye contact, responding with speech, and imitating vocalisations using different patterns and emphasis. For example, raise the pitch of your voice to indicate a question.

- Imitate your baby's laughter and facial expressions.

- Teach your baby to imitate your actions, including clapping your hands, throwing kisses, and playing finger games such as pat-a-cake, peekaboo, and itsy-bitsy-spider.

- Talk as you bathe, feed and dress your baby. Talk about what you are doing, where you are going, what you will do when you arrive, and who and what you will see.

- Identify colours.

- Count items.

- Use gestures such as waving goodbye to help convey meaning.

- Introduce animal sounds to associate a sound with a specific meaning: 'The doggie says woof-woof.'

- Acknowledge the attempt to communicate.

- Expand on single words your baby uses: 'Here is Mama. Mama loves you. Where is baby? Here is baby.'

- Read to your child. Sometimes 'reading' is simply describing the pictures in a book without following the written words. Choose books that are sturdy and have large colourful pictures that are not too detailed. Ask your child, 'What's this?' and encourage naming and pointing to familiar objects in the book.

2 TO 4 YEARS

- Use good speech that is clear and simple for your child to model.

- Repeat what your child says, indicating that you understand. Build and expand on what was said. 'Want juice? I have juice. I have apple juice. Do you want apple juice?'

- Use baby talk only if needed to convey the message and when accompanied by the adult word. 'It is time for din-din. We will have dinner now.'

- Make a scrapbook of favourite or familiar things by cutting out pictures. Group them into categories, such as things to ride on, things to eat, things for dessert, fruits, things to play with. Create silly pictures by mixing and matching pictures. Glue a picture of a dog behind the wheel of a car. Talk about what is wrong with the picture and ways to 'fix' it. Count items pictured in the book.

- Help your child understand and ask questions. Play the yes-no game. Ask questions such as, 'Are you a boy?' 'Are you Marty?' 'Can a pig fly?' Encourage your child to make up questions and try to fool you.

- Ask questions that require a choice. 'Do you want an apple or an orange?' 'Do you want to wear your red or blue shirt?'

- Expand vocabulary. Name body parts, and identify what you do with them. 'This is my nose. I can smell flowers, brownies, popcorn, and soap.'

- Sing simple songs and recite nursery rhymes to show the rhythm and pattern of speech.

- Place familiar objects in a container. Have your child remove the object and tell you what it is called and how to use it. 'This is my ball. I bounce it. I play with it.'

- Use photographs of familiar people and places, and retell what happened or make up a new story.

4 TO 6 YEARS

- When your child starts a conversation, give your full attention whenever possible.

- Make sure that you have your child's attention before you speak.

- Acknowledge, encourage and praise all attempts to speak. Show that you understand the word or phrase by fulfilling the request, if appropriate.

- Pause after speaking. This gives your child a chance to continue the conversation.

- Continue to build vocabulary. Introduce a new word and offer its definition, or use it in a context that is easily understood. This may be done in an exaggerated, humorous manner: 'I think I will drive the vehicle to the store. I am too tired to walk.'

- Talk about spatial relationships (first, middle and last; right and left) and opposites (up and down; on and off).

- Offer a description or clues, and have your child identify what you are describing: 'We use it to sweep the floor' (a broom); 'It is cold, sweet, and good for dessert. I like strawberry' (ice cream).

- Work on forming and explaining categories. Identify the thing that does not belong in a group of similar objects: 'A shoe does not belong with an apple and an orange because you can't eat it; it is not round; it is not a fruit.'

- Help your child follow two- and three-step directions: 'Go to your room, and bring me your book.'

- Encourage your child to give directions. Follow his or her directions as he or she explains how to build a tower of blocks.

- Play games such as 'house' with your child. Exchange roles in the family, with you pretending to be the child. Talk about the different furnishings in the house.

- The television also can serve as a valuable tool. Talk about what the child is watching. Have him or her guess what might happen next. Talk about the characters. Are they happy or sad? Ask your child to tell you what has happened in the story. Act out a scene together, and make up a different ending.

- Take advantage of daily activities. For example, while in the kitchen, encourage your child to name the utensils needed. Discuss the foods on the menu, their colour, texture and taste. Where does the food come from? Which foods do you like? Which do you dislike? Who will clean up? Emphasise the use of prepositions by asking him or her to put the napkin on the table, in your lap, or under the spoon. Identify who the napkin belongs to: 'It is my napkin.' 'It is Daddy's.' 'It is John's.'

- While shopping for groceries, discuss what you will buy, how many you need, and what you will make. Discuss the size (large or small), shape (long, round, square), and weight (heavy or light) of the packages.

A Child's Spirit

Carole Sutton

A child's spirit grows with praise.
Its impact lasts for all his days.
So, if your child's behaving right
Then tell her so with real delight.

Young children don't know right from wrong
They learn it as they go along.
So show them how and tell them why
And praise them then when they comply.

If Mum and Dad and Gran agree
This gives your child security.
So write down rules by shared consent,
They'll save repeated argument.

If misbehaviour's fairly mild
If possible, ignore the child
Ignore complaints and interruptions
Ignore – despite initial ructions!

And if your child is being silly,
Teasing, swearing, shouting 'Willy',
Try to ignore these day by day,
They gradually will fade away.

Deal firmly with your child's request.
Let 'No' mean 'No' and 'Yes' mean 'Yes'.
So if to pester Johnny's learned.
Then turn your back and keep it turned.

But if behaviour's getting wild
You should not then ignore the child.
So fighting, or rude repartee
Calls for a firmer penalty.

A two-year-old who bites or hits
Two minutes in Time Out now sits.
A Time Out place is safe and boring
Very good for child-ignoring.

For little children one to three,
Time Out two minutes long should be.
For older children, please select
Four minutes for the best effect.

If Johnny won't stay in Time Out
But starts to kick and bite and shout,
Check that he's safe – there'll be suspense –
Leave him without an audience.

And if your child plays with his food,
One warning, then it's gone for good.
If 'I don't like this!' is the shout,
Say, 'Very well, then go without'.

If Johnny calls for midnight play,
Don't hurry in; briefly delay,
Then check he's safe; keep calm and cool,
No speech, no eye contact's the rule.

A child's spirit grows with praise,
Its impact lasts for all his days.
So, if your child's behaving right,
Then tell her so with real delight.

Five praises a day

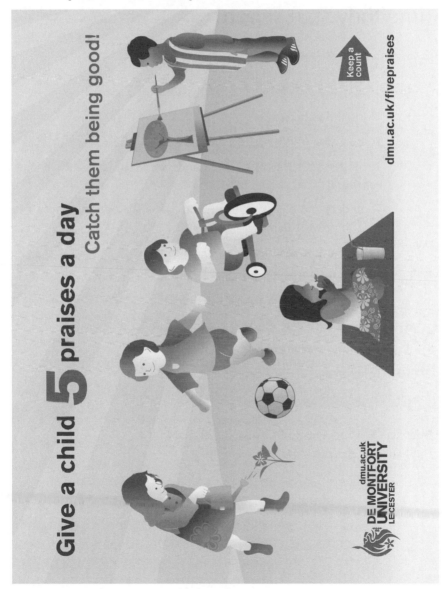

The ten skills a child must have by the time they start school

1. To sit still and listen

2. To be aware of other children

3. To understand the word 'No' and the boundaries it sets for behaviour

4. To understand the word 'Stop' and that such a phrase might be used to prevent danger

5. To be potty trained and able to go to the loo

6. To recognise their own name

7. To speak to an adult to ask for help

8. To be able to take off their coat and put on shoes

9. To talk in sentences

10. To open and enjoy a book

Michael Wilshire, Head of Ofsted, April 2014
Published in the *Daily Mail*

Charting behaviours: doing/not doing as asked

Please tick the number of instances to be used for at least a month.

Behaviour: Does as asked on the first time of asking	Sunday	Monday	Tuesday	Wednesday	Thursday	Friday	Saturday	TOTAL
Morning								
Afternoon								
Evening								

★

Behaviour: Does not do as asked on the first time of asking	Sunday	Monday	Tuesday	Wednesday	Thursday	Friday	Saturday	TOTAL
Morning								
Afternoon								
Evening								

Positive comments to young children

That's really good!

Let's save your drawing to show Granny.

Well done. You've tried so hard.

You've put on your own socks! Great!

You found my missing keys. Hooray!

You've eaten up all your tea. Well done.

You got dressed all by yourself. Wow!

I am very pleased with you for...

You shared the toys with Ann. How kind!

You've worked really hard on that.

That's a fine house you've built.

You came when I called. Thank you.

I like that drawing. Can I pin it up?

Daddy will like that when he comes in.

Yes, wait at the kerb. That's just right.

Yes, stroke the cat carefully... Lovely...

Please help me put the toys away. Fine!

That card will please Grandpa very much.

★

When... then...

When you've put your bike away, then we'll have tea.

When you've washed, and brushed your teeth, then we'll have a story.

When you've done your homework, then you can watch 30 minutes TV.

When you've put this lot of toys away, then you can get out another.

When you've tidied your bedroom, then you can have John round to play.

When you've saved up enough, then you can buy a DVD.

When you've done your jobs, then I'll give you your pocket money.

When the clock shows 8.00 o'clock, then you must go to bed.

When you've hung up your coat, then I'll help you make some pancakes.

When you've cleaned the hamster's cage, then you can go out to play.

APPENDIX 11

Please talk to ME!

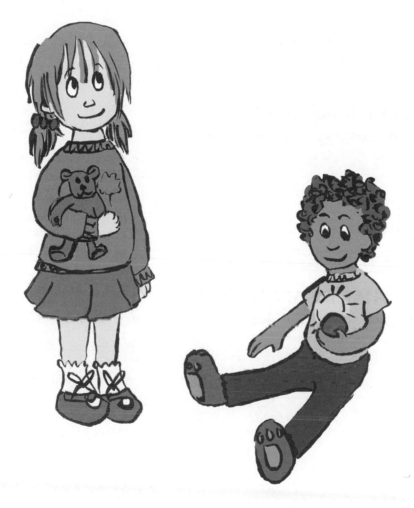

★

Form for framing an agreement in one-to-one or family work

This form is to be completed by the worker in discussion with the young person and family members. It is all-purpose and can be adapted to a range of situations.

A THE AGREEMENT

This agreement is drawn up between:

1 .... 3 ....

2 .... 4 ....

and .... worker from

Agency ....

Address ....

Tel ....

B WHAT WE ARE TRYING TO DO TOGETHER

We have talked about what we can work towards together and agree that our goals are to:

1 ....

2 ....

3 ....

★

C TO WORK TOWARD THESE GOALS

The worker agrees to:

1 ....

2 ....

3 ....

Members of the family agree to:

1st person (name) ....

1..

2..

3..

2nd person (name) ....

1..

2..

3..

3rd person (name) ....

1..

2..

3..

4th person (name) ....

1..

2..

3..

5th person (name) ....

1..

2..

3..

D OTHER POINTS TO BE NOTED

The above agreement is to be reviewed every week/two weeks.

The above agreement can be changed if everyone agrees.

Signed ....

Signed ....

Signed ....

Signed ....

Signed ....

References

Ainsworth, M.D., Bleha, M., Waters, S., and Wall, S. (1978) *Patterns of Attachment. A Psychological Study of the Strange Situation.* Hillsdale, NJ.: Lawrence Erlbaum.

Alexander, J.F., and Parsons, B.V. (1980) *Functional Family Therapy.* Monterey, CA: Brooks Cole Publishing.

Alhusen, J.L. (2008) 'A literature update on maternal-fetal attachment.' *Journal of Obstetric, Gynecologic and Neonatal Nursing 37,* 3, 315–328.

Allen, G. (2011) *Early Intervention: The Next Steps. An Independent Report to Her Majesty's Government* (The Allen Report). London: Cabinet Office.

Anderson, J.W., Johnstone, B.M., and Remley, D.T. (1999) 'Breast-feeding and cognitive development: a meta-analysis.' *American Journal of Clinical Nutrition 70,* 525–535.

Aos, S., Lee, S., Drake, E., Pennucci, A., *et al.* (2011) *Return on Investment. Evidence-based Options to Reduce State-Wide Outcomes* (Document no. 11-07-1201-A). Olympia, WA: Washington State Institute for Public Policy.

Appleyard, K., Egeland, B., van Dulmen, M.H., and Sroufe, L.A. (2005) 'When more is not better: the role of cumulative risk in child behavior outcomes.' *Journal of Child Psychology and Psychiatry 46,* 3, 235–245.

Asay, T.P., and Lambert, M.J. (1999) 'The Empirical Case for the Common Factors in Therapy. Quantitative Findings.' In M.A. Hubble, B.L. Duncan and S.D. Miller (eds) *The Heart and Soul of Change.* Washington, D.C.: American Psychological Association.

Bakermans-Kranenburg, M.J., van Ijzendoorn, M.H. and Juffer, F. (2003). 'Less is more: Meta-analyses of sensitivity and attachment interventions in early childhood.' *Psychological Bulletin, 129,* 195-215.

Baumrind, D. (1971) 'Current patterns of parental authority.' *Developmental Psychology Monographs 1,* 1–102.

Beckett, C., Beecham, J., Doolan, M., Ford, T., *et al.*, with the HCA Study Teams (2012) 'Which type of parenting programme best improves child behaviour and reading?' *The Helping Children Achieve Trial* (DFE-RR261). London: Department for Education.

Berger, P.L. (1966) *Invitation to Sociology.* Harmondsworth: Penguin.

Berk, L. (2006) *Child Development* (7th edition). Boston, MA: Pearson International Edition.

Bicking-Kinsey, C., and Hupcey, J. (2013) 'State of the science of maternal-infant bonding: a principle-based concept analysis.' *Midwifery 29*, 12, 1314–1320.

Bidmead, C., and Andrews, L. (2004) 'Enhancing early parent-infant interaction. Part one: Observations strategies.' *Community Practitioner 77*, 10, 187–189.

Bidmead, C., and Mackinder, L. (2004) 'Enhancing early parent-infant interaction. Part three: Early play.' *Community Practitioner 77*, 12, 471–473.

Blair, J., Mitchell, D., and Blair, K. (2005) *The Psychopath: Emotion and the Brain*. Oxford. Blackwell.

Blaze, J.T., Olmi, D.J., Mercer, S., Dufrene, B., and Tingstom, D.H. (2014) 'Loud versus quiet praise: a direct behavioral comparison in secondary classrooms.' *Journal of School Psychology 52*, 349–360.

Bonyata, K. (2011) *Encouraging Teen Moms to Breastfeed*. Available at http://kellymom. com/pregnancy/bf-prep/teenbf, accessed on 22 September 2015.

Bowlby, J. (1979) *The Making and Breaking of Affectional Bonds*. London: Tavistock.

Boyce, L. (2014) *Pocket Money is the Key to Strong Financial Skills in Later Life*. Available at www.thisismoney.co.uk/money/saving/article-2749431/Pocket-money-key-strong-financial-skills-later-life.html, accessed on 22 September 2015.

Bradley, R., Corwyn, R., McAdoo, H., and Garcia Coll, C. (2001) 'The home environments of children in the United States.' *Child Development 72*, 1844–1867.

Brayne, H., and Carr, H. (2008) *Law for Social Workers* (10th edition) Oxford: Oxford University Press.

Brazelton, T.B., and Nugent, J.K. (1995) *The Neonatal Behavioral Assessment Scale*. London: McKeith Press.

Brockington, I. (2001) 'A screening questionnaire for mother-infant bonding disorders.' *Archives of Women's Mental Health 3*, 133–140.

Bunn, A. (2013) Signs of Safety in England. An NSPCC Commissioned Report on the Signs of Safety Model in Child Protection. NSPCC. London.

Burnette, M.L., Oshri, A., Lax, R., Richards, D., and Ragbeer, S.N. (2012) 'Pathways from harsh parenting to adolescent antisocial behavior: a multidomain test of gender moderation.' *Developmental Psychopathology 24*, 3, 857–870.

Carr, A. (2004) *Positive Psychology: The Science of Happiness and Human Strengths*. London. Routledge.

Caspi, A, Taylor, A., Moffitt, T.E., and Plomin, R. (2000) 'Neighbourhood deprivation affects children's mental health: environmental risks identified in a genetic design.' *Psychological Science 11*, 338–342.

Cheminais, R. (2009) *Effective Multi-Agency Partnerships: Putting Every Child Matters into Practice*. London: Department for Education.

Cheng, C.D., Volk, A.A., and Marini, Z.M. (2011) 'Supporting fathering through infant massage.' *Journal of Perinatal Education 20*, 4, 200–209.

Coleman, J., and Hendry, L. (2000) *The Nature of Adolescence* (3rd edition). London: Routledge.

Cox, J., Holden, J., and Sagovsky, R. (1987) 'Detection of postnatal depression. Development of the 10-Item Edinburgh Postnatal Depression Scale.' *British Journal of Psychiatry 159*, 782–786.

Deklyen, M., and Speltz, M.I. (2001) 'Attachment and Conduct Disorder.' In J. Hill and B. Maughan (eds) *Conduct Disorders in Childhood and Adolescence.* Cambridge: Cambridge University Press.

Department for Education (2003) *Every Child Matters.* Norwich: The Stationery Office.

Department for Education (2011) *The Early Years: Foundation for Life, Health and Learning. An Independent Report on the Early Years Foundation Stage to Her Majesty's Government.* London: The Stationery Office.

Department for Education (2013) *Early Years Foundation Stage Profile by Pupil Characteristics. England.* London: Department for Education.

Department for Education (2014a) *Characteristics of Children in Need in England, 2013– 2014.* Statistical first release SFR43/2014. London: Department for Education.

Department for Education (2014b) *National Curriculum Assessments at Key Stage 2 in England 2014 (Revised).* Statistical First Release. London: Department for Education.

Department for Education (2015) *Working Together to Safeguard Children. A Guide to Inter- Agency Working to Safeguard and Promote the Welfare of Children.* London: Department for Education.

Department of Health (2000) *Framework for the Assessment of Children in Need and their Families.* London: HMSO.

Department of Health (2011) *Off to the Best Start. Important Information About Feeding Your Baby.* London: Department of Health.

Dilmore, D.L. (2004) *A Comparison of Confidence Levels Between Postpartum Depressed and Non-Depressed First Time Mothers.* Electronic Theses, Treatises and Dissertations, Florida State University, Paper 84. Available at http://diginole.lib.fsu.edu/cgi/viewcontent.cgi?article=1210&context=etd, accessed on 22 September 2015.

Dunkel Schetter, C., and Tanner, I. (2012) 'Anxiety, depression and stress in pregnancy: implications for mothers, children, research and practice.' *Current Opinion in Psychiatry 25*, 2, 141–148.

Duursma, E., Augustyn, M., and Zuckerman, B. (2008) 'Reading aloud to children: the evidence.' *Archives of Disease in Childhood 93*, 554–557.

Eckenrode, J., Campa, M., Luckey, D., Henderson, C., *et al.* (2010) 'Long-term effects of prenatal and infancy nurse home visitation on the life course of youths: 19-year follow-up of a randomized trial.' *Archives of Pediatric and Adolescent Medicine 164*, 9–15.

Fahlberg, V. (1988) *Fitting the Pieces Together.* London: British Association for Adoption and Fostering.

Fall, K.A., Miner Holden, J., and Marquis, A. (2004) *Theoretical Models of Counseling and Psychotherapy.* Hove: Brunner-Routledge.

Farrington, D., and Coid, J.W. (eds) (2003) *Early Prevention of Adult Antisocial Behaviour.* Cambridge: Cambridge University Press.

Feldman, R., Weller, A., Zagoory-Sharon, O., *et al.* (2007) 'Evidence for a neuroendocrinological foundation of human affiliation: plasma oxytocin levels across pregnancy and the postpartum period predict mother-infant bonding.' *Psychological Science 18*, 11, 965–970.

Ferguson, H.B., Bovaird, M.P.H., and Mueller, M.P. (2007) 'The impact of poverty on educational outcomes for children.' *Paediatrics and Child Health 12*, 8, 701–706.

Fergusson, D.M., Horwood, L.J., and Ridder, E.M. (2005) 'Show me the child at seven: the consequences of conduct problems in childhood for psychosocial functioning in adulthood.' *Journal of Child Psychology and Psychiatry 46*, 837–849.

Field, T., Diego, M., and Hernando-Reif, M. (2010) 'Preterm infant massage therapy research. A review.' *Infant Behaviour Development 33*, 2, 115–134.

Flach, C., Leese, M., Heron, J., *et al.* (2011) 'Antenatal domestic violence, maternal mental health and subsequent child behaviour: a cohort study.' *BJOG 118*, 11, 1383–1391.

Fluckiger, C., and Grosse Holtforth, M. (2008) -Focusing the therapist's attention on the patient's strengths: a preliminary study to foster a mechanism of change in outpatient psychotherapy.' *Journal of Clinical Psychology 64*, 7, 876–890.

Fox, K. (n.d) '10 ways to get active with your kid.' Available at www.nhs.uk/Livewell/childhealth6-15/Pages/Getactivewithyourkids.aspx, accessed on 16 November 2015.

Ghate, D., and Ramella, M. (2002) *Positive Parenting. The National Evaluation of the Youth Justice Board's Parenting Programme.* London: Youth Justice Board.

Goldberg, D.P, Cooper, B., Eastwood, M.R., Kedward, H.B., and Shepherd, M. (1970) 'A standardised psychiatric interview for use in community settings.' *British Journal of Preventive and Social Medicine 24*,1, 18–23.

Goodman, R. (1997) 'The Strengths and Difficulties Questionnaire: A Research Note.' *Journal of Child Psychology and Psychiatry, 5*, 581–586.

Goodwyn, S.W., Acredolo, L., and Brown, C.A. (2000) 'Impact of symbolic gesturing on early language development.' *Journal of Nonverbal Behaviour 24*, 81–103.

Government of Western Australia (2011) *The Signs of Safety: Child Protection Practice Framework.* East Perth, WA 6004: Department of Child Protection.

Grant, K., O'Koon, J., Davis, T., Roache, N., Poindexter, L., and Armstrong, M. (2000) 'Protective factors affecting low-income urban African American youth exposed to stress.' *Journal of Early Adolescence 20*, 388–418.

Grossman, J.B., and Tierney, J.P. (1998) 'Does mentoring work? An evaluation of the Big Brothers Big Sisters program.' *Evaluation Review 22*, 3, 403–426.

Hart, B., and Risley, T.R. (1995) *Meaningful Differences in the Everyday Experience of Young American Children.* London: Brookes.

He, H.L., Yan, H., Zuo, L., Liu, L., and Zhang, X.P. (2009) 'Effects of Montessori education on the intellectual development in children aged 2 to 4 years.' *Zhongguo Dang Dai Er Ke Za Zhi 11*, 12, 1002–1005.

Henggeler, S.W, Schoenwald, S.K., Borduin, C.M., Rowland, M., and Cunningham, P.B. (1998) *Multisystemic Treatment of Antisocial Behaviour in Children and Adolescents.* New York: Guilford Press.

Herbert, M. (1987) *Behavioural Treatment of Children with Problems.* London: Academic Press.

Herbert, M., Sluckin, V., and Sluckin, A. (1982) 'Mother-to-infant bonding.' *Journal of Child Psychology and Psychiatry 2,* 3, 205–221.

Hoeve, M., Dubas, J., Eichelsheim, V., van der Laan, P.H., Smeenk, W., and Gerris, J.R. (2009) 'The relationship between parenting and delinquency: a meta-analysis.' *Journal of Abnormal Child Psychology 37,* 6, 749–775.

Holden, J., Sagovsky, R., and Cox, J. (1989) 'Counselling in a general practice setting: controlled study of health visitor intervention in treatment of postnatal depression.' *British Medical Journal 298,* 223–226.

Howe, M. (1990) *Sense and Nonsense about Hot House Children: a Practical Guide for Parents.* Leicester: British Psychological Society.

Jolliffe, D., and Farrington, D.P. (2007) *A Rapid Evidence Assessment of the Impact of Mentoring on Re-Offending: a Summary.* Home Office Online Report 11/07. Available at www.crim.cam.ac.uk/people/academic_research/david_farrington/olr1107. pdf, accessed on 22 September 2015.

Joosen, K.J., Mesman, J., Bakermans-Kranenberg, M.J., *et al.* (2012) 'Maternal sensitivity to infants in various settings predicts harsh discipline in toddlerhood.' *Attachment and Human Development 14,* 2, 101–117.

Keefe, M.R., Froese-Fretz, A., and Kefzer, A.M. (1997) 'The REST regime; an individualized nursing intervention for infant irritability.' *American Journal of Maternal Nursing 22,* 16–20.

Kennell J., and McGrath, S. (2005) 'Starting the process of mother-infant bonding.' *Acta Paediactrica 94,* 6, 775–777.

Kochanska, G. (1993) 'Toward a synthesis of parental socialization and child temperament in early development of conscience.' *Child Development 64,* 325–347.

Lane, E., Gardner, F., Hutchings, J., and Jacobs, B. (2004) 'Nine to 13 Years: Risk and Protective Factors; Effective Interventions.' In C. Sutton, D. Utting and D. Farrington (eds) *Support from the Start.* RR 524. Nottingham: DfES Publications.

Latendresse, G. (2009) 'The interaction between chronic stress and pregnancy: preterm birth from a biobehavioral perspective.' *Journal of Midwifery and Women's Health 54,* 1, 8–17.

Lee, G.Y., and Kisilevsky, B. (2014) 'Fetuses respond to father's voice but prefer mother's voice after birth.' *Developmental Psychobiology 56,* 1, 1–11.

Loeber, R., and Stouthamer-Loeber, M. (1986) 'Family Factors as Correlates and Predictors of Juvenile Conduct Problems and Delinquency.' In M.H. Tonry and H. Morris (eds) *Crime and Justice. An Annual Review of Research, Vol. 7.* Chicago: University of Chicago Press.

Lyons-Ruth, K. (1996) 'Attachment relationships among children with aggressive behaviour problems. The role of disorganized early attachment patterns.' *Journal of Consulting and Clinical Psychology 64*, 64–73.

Lyons-Ruth, K., Bronfman, E., and Parsons, E. (1999) 'Maternal frightened, frightening or atypical behaviour and disorganized infant attachment patterns.' *Monographs of the Society for Research in Child Development 64*, 3, Serial no. 258, 67–96.

Maccoby, E., and Martin, J.A. (1983) 'Socialisation in the Context of the Family: Parent-Child Interaction.' In P.H. Mussen (ed.) *Handbook of Child Psychology, Vol. 4*. Chichester: Wiley.

Mackenzie, M.J., Nicklas, E., Brooks-Gunn, J., and Waldfogel, J. (2011) 'Who spanks infants and toddlers? Evidence from the fragile families and child well-being study.' *Child and Youth Service Review 33*, 8, 1364–1373.

MacKenzie, M.J., Nicklas, E., Waldfogel, J., and Brooks-Gunn, J. (2012) 'Corporal punishment and child behavioral and cognitive outcomes through five years-of-age. Evidence from a contemporary urban birth cohort study.' *Infant and Child Development 21*, 1, 1–33.

Main, M., and Soloman, J. (1986) 'Discovery of an Insecure Disorganised/Disorientated Attachment Pattern: Procedures, Findings and Implications for the Classification of Behaviour.' In B. Brazelton and M. Yogman (eds) *Affective Development in Infancy*. Norwood, NJ: Ablex.

Mann, R., Adamson, J., and Gilbody, S. (2012) 'Diagnostic accuracy of case-finding questions to identify perinatal depression.' *Canadian Medical Association Journal 184*, 8, E424–E430.

Mares, P., Henley, A., and Baxter, C. (1985) *Health Care in Multiracial Britain*. London: Health Education Council/National Extension College.

Martin, C., and Pear, J. (1992) *Behavior Modification. What It Is and How To Do It*. Prentice Hall: Hemel Hempstead.

McCourt, C., and Pearce, A. (2000) 'Does continuity of care matter to women in minority ethnic groups?' *Midwifery 16*, 2, 145–154.

McCourt, C., Stevens, T., Sandall, J., and Brodie, P. (2006) 'Working With Women: Developing Continuity of Care in Practice.' In L.A. Page and R. McCandlish (eds) *The New Midwifery*. London: Churchill Livingstone Elsevier.

Milgrom, J., Gemmill, A., Ericksen, J., Burrows, G., *et al.* (2015) 'Treatment of postnatal depression with cognitive behavioural therapy, sertraline and combination therapy: a randomised controlled trial.' *Australian and New Zealand Journal of Psychiatry 49*, 3, 236–245.

Mindell, J.A., Telofski, L.S., Wiegand, Kurtz, E.S. (2009) 'A Nightly Bedtime Routine: Impact on Sleep in Young Children and Maternal Mood.' *SLEEP 2009, 32*, 5, 599–606.

Mischel, W., Mishoda, Y., and Rodriguez, M. (1989) 'Delay of gratification in children.' *Science 244*, 933–938.

Moffitt, T., Arseneault, L., Belsky, D., Dickson, N., *et al.* (2011) 'A gradient of childhood self control predicts health, wealth and public safety.' *Proceedings of the National Academy of Sciences 108*, 7, 2693–2698.

Moffitt, T.E. (1993) 'Adolescence-limited and life-course-persistent antisocial behavior. A developmental taxonomy.' *Psychological Review 100*, 674–701.

Mohr, W., and Anderson, J.A. (2002) 'Reconsidering punitive and harsh discipline.' *Journal of School Nursing 18*, 6, 346–352.

National Evaluation of Sure Start Research Team (NESS) (2008) *The Impact of Sure Start Local Programmes on Seven Year Olds and Their Families.* Research report DFE-RR220. London: Department for Education.

National Foundation for Educational Research (NFER) (2015) *Progress in International Reading Literacy Study.* Available at www.nfer.ac.uk/research/projects/progress-in-reading-literacy-study-pirls, accessed on 22 September 2015.

National Institute for Health and Care Excellence (NICE) Local Government Briefing (2013) *Social and Emotional Wellbeing for Children and Young People. Available at* http://publications.nice.org.uk/lgb12, accessed on 22 September 2015.

Newton, N., Andrews, G., Teesson, M., and Vogl, L. (2009) 'Delivering prevention for alcohol and cannabis using the internet: a cluster randomised controlled trial.' *Preventive Medicine 48*, 6, 579–584.

NHS England (2014) *Child and Adolescent Mental Health Services (CAMHS) Tier 4 Report.* London: NHS England.

Nikolopoulou, M., and St. James-Roberts, I. (2003) 'Preventing sleeping problems in infants who are at risk of developing them.' *Archives of Disease in Childhood 88*, 108–111.

Nugent, J.K. (1985) *Using the Neonatal Behavioral Assessment Scale with Infants and their Families.* White Plains, New York: March of Dimes Birth Defects Foundation.

Nugent, J.K., Keefer, C., Minear, S., Johnson, L., and Blanchard, Y. (2007) *Understanding Newborn Behavior and Early Relationships. The Newborn Behavioural Observations (NBO) System Handbook.* Baltimore: Paul H. Brookes.

O'Connor, R., and Waddell, S. (2015) *Preventing Gang Involvement and Youth Violence. Advice for those Commissioning Mentoring Programmes.* London: Home Office/Early Intervention Foundation.

O'Connor, T.G., Heron, J., Golding, J., Beveridge, M., and Glover, V. (2002) 'Maternal antenatal anxiety and children's behavioural/emotional problems at 4 years. Report from the Avon Longitudinal Study of Parents and Children.' *British Journal of Psychiatry 180*, 502–508.

Odgers, C. L., Caspi, A., Russell, M., Sampson, R., Arsenault, L., and Moffitt, T.E. (2012) 'Supportive parenting mediates widening neighborhood socioeconomic disparities in children's antisocial behavior from ages 5 to 12.' *Development and Psychopathology 24*, 3, 705–721.

Ofsted (2014) *Are You Ready? Good Practice in School Readiness.* Manchester: Ofsted. Crown Copyright.

Olds, D., *et al.* (1998) 'Long-term effects of nurse home visitation on children's criminal and antisocial behavior.' *Journal of the American Medical Association 80*, 1238–1244.

Paradis, A.D., Fitzmaurice, G.M., Koenen, K.C., and Buka, S. (2011) 'Maternal smoking during pregnancy and criminal offending among adult offspring.' *Journal of Epidemiology and Community Health 65*, 12, 1145–1150.

Patterson, G.R. (1976) *Living with Children. New Methods for Parents and Teachers.* Champaign, IL: Research Press.

Perra, O., Fletcher, A., Bonell, C. Higgins, K., and McCrystal, P. (2012) 'School-related predictors of smoking, drinking and drug use: evidence from the Belfast Youth Development Study.' *Journal of Adolescence 35*, 2, 315–324.

Protzko, J., Aronson, J., and Blair, C. (2013) 'How to make a young child smarter: evidence from the database of raising intelligence.' *Perspectives on Psychological Science 8*, 25–40.

Public Health England (2015) *Rapid Review to Update Evidence for the Healthy Child Programme 0–5.* London: Department of Health.

Ramchandani, P.G., Domoney, J., Sethna, V., Psychogiou, L., Vlachos, H., and Murray, L. (2013) 'Do early father-infant interactions predict the onset of externalizing behaviours in young children? Findings from a longitudinal cohort study.' *Journal of Child Psychology and Psychiatry 54*, 1, 56–64.

Redshaw, M., and Henderson, J. (2013) 'Fathers' engagement in pregnancy and childbirth: evidence from a national survey.' *BMC Pregnancy and Childbirth 13*, 70.

Reid, J.B., and Patterson, G.R. (1989) 'The development of antisocial patterns of behavior in childhood and adolescence.' *European Journal of Personality 3*, 107–119.

Robins, L.N. (1966) *Deviant Children Grown Up. A Sociological and Psychiatric Study of Sociopathic Personality.* Baltimore, MD: Williams and Wilkins.

Rogers, C. (1951) *Client Centred Therapy.* Boston: Houghton-Mifflin.

Rohner, R., and Veneziano, R. (2001) 'The importance of father love: history and contemporary evidence.' *Review of General Psychology 5*, 382–405.

Rollnick, S., Miller, W., and Butler, C.C. (2008) *Motivational Interviewing in Health Care.* London: Guilford.

Rowan, C., Doan, A., and Cash, H. (2014) *Technology Use Guidelines for Children and Youth.* Available at: www.huffingtonpost.com/cris-rowan/10-reasons-why-handheld-devices-should-be-banned_b_4899218.html, accessed on 16 November 2015.

Rutter, M. (1978) 'Family and School Influences in the Genesis of Conduct Disorders.' In L.A. Hersov, M. Berger and D. Shaffer (eds) *Aggression and Antisocial Behaviour in Childhood and Adolescence.* Oxford: Pergamon.

Rutter, M., Giller, H., and Hagell, A. (1998) *Antisocial Behavior by Young People.* Cambridge: Cambridge University Press.

Rutter, M., Maughan, B., Mortimore, P., Ouston, J., and Smith, A. (1979) *Fifteen Thousand Hours. Secondary Schools and Their Effects on Children.* Cambridge, MA: Harvard University Press.

Saleebey, D. (2005) *The Strengths Perspective in Social Work Practice.* London: Allyn and Bacon/Longman.

Sanders, M.R. (1999) 'Triple P-Positive Parenting Program: towards an empirically validated multilevel parenting and family support strategy for the prevention of behavior and emotional problems in children.' *Clinical Child and Family Psychology Review 2*, 2, 71–90.

Sanders, M.R. (1999) Triple P-Positive Parenting Program: towards an empirically validated multilevel parenting and family support strategy for the prevention of behavior and emotional problems in children. *Clinical Child and Family Psychology Review*, 2, 2, 71-90.

Sarkadi, A., Kristiansson, R., Oberklaid, F. and Bremberg, S. (2008) Fathers' involvement and children's developmental outcomes: a systematic review of longitudinal studies. *Acta Paediatrica*, 97, 154–158.

Scope, A., Leavis, J., Kaltenthaler, E., Parry, G., Sutcliffe, P., Bradburn, M. and Cantrell, A. (2013), Is group cognitive behavior therapy for postnatal depression evidence-based practice? A systematic review. *BMC Psychiatry*, 13, 321. doi:10.1186/1471-244X-13-321.

Scott S., Doolan, M., Beckett C., Harry, S., Cartwright, S., and HCA team (2012) *Helping Children Achieve.* London: Department for Education.

Scott, S. (2006) 'Improving children's lives: preventing criminality: Where next?' *The Psychologist 19*, 8, 484–487.

Scott, S., Sylva, K., Kallitsoglou, A., and Ford, T. (2014) *Which Type of Parenting Programme Best Improves Child Behaviour and Reading? Follow-up of the Helping Children Achieve Trial.* London. Nuffield Foundation.

Selwyn, J., Wijedasa, D., and Meakings, S., University of Bristol School for Policy Studies (2014) *Beyond the Adoption Order. Challenges, Intervention and Adoption Disruption.* London: Department for Education.

Sharma, A., and Cockerill, H. (2014) *Mary Sheridan's From Birth to Five Years. Children's Developmental Progress* (4th edition). London: Routledge.

Sharp, D.J., Chew-Graham, C., Tylee, A., Lewis, G., *et al.* (2010) 'A pragmatic randomised controlled trial to compare antidepressants with a community-based psychosocial intervention for the treatment of women with postnatal depression: the RESPOND trial.' *Health Technology Assessment 14*, 43, iii–iv, ix–xi, 1–153.

Sheldon, B. (1980) *The Use of Contracts in Social Work.* Birmingham: British Association of Social Workers.

Sheridan, M. (2008) *From Birth to Five years. Children's Developmental Progress* (3rd edition, revised and updated by A. Sharma and H. Cockerill). London: Routledge.

Silverstein, D. (1996) *Specific techniques to increase family attachment.* Available at www.adopting.org/silveroze/html/attachment.html.

Spivack, C., Platt, J.J., and Shure, M. (1976) *The Problem-Solving Approach to Adjustment.* San Francisco, CA: Jossey-Bass.

Steele, M. L., Marigna, M.K., Tello, J. and Johnson, R. (1999) Strengthening multi-ethnic families and communities: A violence prevention parent training program. Los Angeles, C.A.: Consulting and Clinical Services. Stevenson, J., and Goodman,

R. (2001) 'Association between behaviour at age 3 years and adult criminality.' *British Journal of Psychiatry 179*, 197–202.

Sutton, C. (1992) 'Training parents to manage difficult children: a comparison of methods.' *Behavioural Psychotherapy 20*, 115–139.

Sutton, C. (1995) 'Parent training by telephone: a partial replication.' *Behavioural and Cognitive Psychotherapy 23*, 1–24.

Sutton, C. (2001) 'Resurgence of attachment (behaviours) within a cognitive behavioural intervention: evidence from research.' *Behavioural and Cognitive Psychotherapy 29*, 357–366.

Sutton, C. (2006) *Helping Families with Troubled Children. A Preventive Approach* (2nd edition). Chichester: Wiley.

Sutton, C., and Glover, V. (2004) 'Pregnancy: risk and protective factors; effective interventions.' In C. Sutton, D. Utting and D. Farrington (eds). Support from the Start. London: DfES.

Sutton, C., and Hampton, D. (2013) *Parenting Positively*. Leicester: De Montfort University.

Sutton, C. and Herbert, M. (1992) Mental Health: a Client Support Resource Pack. Windsor: National Foundation for Educational Research, Nelson.

Sutton, C., and Herbert, M. (2008) 'Five praises a day. A proactive approach to encourage good mental health.' *Community Practitioner 81*, 4, 19–22.

Sutton, C., Utting, D., and Farrington, D. (eds) (2004) *Support from the Start. Working with Young Children and Their Families to Reduce the Risks of Crime and Antisocial Behaviour.* RR 524. London: DfES.

Sylva, K., Melhuish, E., Sammons, P., Siraj-Blatchford, I. and Taggart, B. (2004) *The Effective Provision of Pre-School Education (EPPE) Project. Findings from Pre-school to end of Key Stage 1. Research Brief.* DfES Publications: Nottingham.

Taylor, T., and Biglan, A. (1998) 'Behavioural family interventions for improving child-rearing: a review for clinicians and policy makers.' *Clinical Child and Family Psychology Review 1*, 41–60.

Thompson, N. (2006) *Anti-Discriminatory Practice*. Basingstoke: Palgrave Macmillan.

Tolan, P., Henry, D., Schoeny, M., and Bass, A. (2008) 'School-based mentoring for adolescents: a systematic review and meta-analysis.' *Research on Social Work Practice 22*, 3, 257–269.

Tronick, E., and Cohn, J.F. (1989) 'Infant-mother face-to-face interaction: age and gender differences in coordination and the occurrence of miscoordination.' *Child Development 60*, 1, 85–92.

Tronick, E., and Reck, C. (2009) 'Infants of depressed mothers.' *Harvard Review of Psychiatry 17*, 2, 147–156.

Truax, C., and Carkhuff, R. (1967) *Towards Effective Counselling and Psychotherapy.* Chicago: Aldine.

Turck, D. (2005) 'Breast feeding: health benefits for child and mother.' *Archives de Pediatrie 12*, Supple 3, S145–165.

Turnell, A. and Edwards, S. (1999) Signs of Safety: A Solution and Safety Oriented Approach to Child Protection Casework. New York: Norton.

Underdown, A., Barlow, J., Chung, V., and Stewart-Brown, S. (2006) 'Massage intervention for promoting mental and physical health in infants aged under six months.' *Cochrane Database of System Reviews 4*, CD005038.

UNICEF UK (2013) *The Evidence and Rationale for the UNICEF UK Baby Friendly Initiative standards.* London: UNICEF.

Veneziano, R.A. (2003) 'The importance of paternal warmth.' *Cross-Cultural Research 37*, 265–281.

Verlinden, M., Tiemeier, H., Hudziak, J.J., Jaddoe, V.W., *et al.* (2012) 'Television viewing and externalizing problems in preschool children. The Generation R Study.' *Archives of Pediatric and Adolescent Medicine 166*, 10, 919–925.

Viding, E. (2004) 'Annotation: understanding the development of psychopathy.' *Journal of Child Psychology and Psychiatry 45*, 1329–1337.

Wade, S.L., Walz, N.C., Carey, J., McMullen, K., *et al.* (2011) 'Effect on behavior problems of teen online problem-solving for adolescent traumatic brain injury.' *Pediatrics 128*, 4, 947–953.

Webster-Stratton C, Rinaldi J, Jamila MR (2011) Long-Term Outcomes of Incredible Years Parenting Program: Predictors of Adolescent Adjustment. *Child and Adolescent Mental Health., 16*, 1, 38–46.

Webster-Stratton, C. (1992) *The Incredible Years. A Trouble-Shooting Guide for Parents of Children aged 3-8.* Toronto: Umbrella Press.

Whooley, M.A., Avins, A., Miranda, J., and Browner, W.S. (1997) 'Case-finding instruments for depression. Two questions are as good as many.' *Journal of General Internal Medicine 12*, 7, 439–445.

Widarsson, M., Engstrom, G., Tyden, T., Lundberg, P., and Hammar, L.M. (2015) '"Paddling upstream": fathers' involvement during pregnancy as described by expectant fathers and mothers.' *Journal of Clinical Nursing 24*, 7–8, 1059–1068.

Widarsson, M., Kerstis, B., Sundquist, K., Engstrom, G., and Sarkadi, A. (2012) 'Support needs of expectant mothers and fathers: a qualitative study.' *Journal of Perinatal Education 21*, 1, 36–44.

Wilkes, L., Mannix, J., and Jackson, D. (2012) '"I am going to be a dad": experiences and expectations of adolescent and young adult expectant fathers.' *Journal of Clinical Nursing 21*, 1–2, 180–188.

Willson, R., and Branch, R. (2006) *Cognitive Behavioural Therapy for Dummies.* Chichester: Wiley.

Wilson, H. (1980) 'Parental supervision: a neglected aspect of delinquency.' *British Journal of Criminology 20*, 203–235.

Wilson, H. (1987) 'Parental supervision re-examined.' *British Journal of Criminology 27*, 275–301.

Zald, D. (2003) 'The human amygdala and the emotional evaluation of sensory stimuli.' *Brain Research Reviews 41*, 1, 88–123.

Zimmerman, F.J., and Christakis, D.A. (2005) 'Children's television viewing and cognitive outcomes: a longitudinal analysis of national data.' *Archives of Pediatric*

SUBJECT INDEX

AUTHOR INDEX

A Practical Guide to Early Intervention and Family Support

Assessing Needs and Building Resilience in Families Affected by Parental Mental Health and Substance Misuse

Emma Sawyer and Sheryl Burton

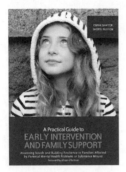

Paperback: £22.99 / $39.95
ISBN: 978 1 90939 121 5
eISBN: 978 1 90939 130 7
288 pages

Parental mental health problems and substance misuse affect a significant number of families. This handbook provides practitioners with early intervention techniques and effective support strategies for ensuring the best outcomes for these vulnerable families.

Featuring pointers, models and practice examples, *A Practical Guide to Early Intervention and Family Support* considers the concept of resilience and effective family support. Assessing the policy context and possible barriers to support, it looks at assessment of need, safeguarding children, minimising negative impact, and most importantly, keeping families together where possible. Drawing on key research on the risks and impacts, this book demonstrates the need for a unified approach from a range of adult and children's services. This third edition has been fully updated to reflect developments in policy and services.

Essential reading for all professionals who are involved in providing services to families, it will also be of interest to service commissioners and those with an academic interest in what helps to support children and families in these circumstances.

Emma Sawyer has worked as a social worker, manager and trainer, she has extensive experience of working with children and families with complex and challenging needs. Whilst working for National Children's Bureau, Emma published several resources on how services can best work together to support parenting more effectively.

Sheryl Burton is Programme Director of National Children's Bureau's Health and Social Care programme. Prior to joining NCB, Sheryl worked as a social work practitioner and team leader, specialising in work with children and families on the threshold of care. Sheryl has extensive experience of working with frontline practitioners and services to develop practice to support children and families more effectively and has written a number of publications for NCB.

Social Work with Troubled Families
A Critical Introduction
Edited by Keith Davies

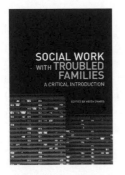

Paperback: £22.99 / $39.95
ISBN: 978 1 84905 549 9
eISBN: 978 0 85700 974 6
192 pages

A critical introduction to the Troubled Families Programme (TFP), this book explores the roots, significance and effectiveness of troubled family approaches in social work.

An important strand of government social policy, the TFP gives rise to a number of ethical and political questions about assertive outreach, choice, use of power and eliding the structural inequalities which, it is often argued, largely account for the difficulties troubled families face. Social Work with Troubled Families: A Critical Introduction debates these issues, offers an examination of the systemic framework which underpins it and looks at the initiative in a broader context.

This interdisciplinary study will be an important resource for social workers, social work students, practice educators and academics for its examination of practice methods. As an exploration of social policy it will appeal to social scientists and to policy makers along with those who seek to influence them.

Keith Davies BA, MSc, MRes is Associate Professor at Kingston University. He has many years of experience working with 'troubled families', largely as a practitioner in criminal justice. Keith has had articles published in The Probation Journal, The Journal of Social Work Education and the British Journal of Community Justice.

Working with Children and Teenagers Using Solution Focused Approaches
Enabling Children to Overcome Challenges and Achieve their Potential
Judith Milner and Jackie Bateman

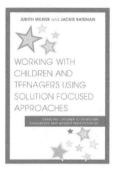

Paperback: £19.99 / $34.95

ISBN: 978 1 84905 082 1

eISBN: 978 0 85700 261 7

176 pages

Solution focused approaches offer proven ways of helping children overcome a whole range of difficulties, from academic problems to mental health issues, by helping them to identify their strengths and achievements.

Based on solution focused practice principles, this book illustrates communication skills and playful techniques for working with all children and young people, regardless of any health, learning or development need. It demonstrates how the approach can capture children's views, wishes and worries, and can assist them in identifying their strengths and abilities. The approach encourages positive decision-making, and helps children to overcome challenges, achieve their goals and reach their full potential. The book is packed with case examples, practical strategies, and practice activities.

This valuable text will be of great use to a range of practitioners working with children and young people, including social workers, youth workers, counsellors, teachers and nurses.

Judith Milner and **Jackie Bateman** are both solution focused practitioners, trainers, consultants and writers. Previously a senior lecturer in social work, Judith now acts as an a therapist, consultant and Independent Expert to family courts in child protection, domestic violence and contested contact cases.